THE

OIL

THAT

HEALS

THE

OIL

THAT

HEALS

A Physician's Successes with Castor Oil Treatments

(Expanded and revised edition of
Edgar Cayce and the Palma Christi)

by William A. McGarey, M.D.

A.R.E. Press • Virginia Beach • Virginia

A.R.E. Press
Sixty-Eighth & Atlantic Avenue
P.O. Box 656
Virginia Beach, VA 23451-0656

Library of Congress Cataloging-in-Publication Data
McGarey, William A., 1919-
    The oil that heals : a physician's successes with castor oil treat-
ments / by William A. McGarey.
    p. cm.
    Expanded and rev. ed. of: Edgar Cayce and the Palma Christi.
    Includes bibliographical references.
    ISBN 0-87604-308-2
    1. Castor oil—Therapeutic use . 2. Cayce, Edgar, 1877-
1945. I. McGarey, William A. Edgar Cayce and the Palma
Christi. II. Title.
RM666.C375M38 1993
615'.32395—dc20   93-26185

Cover illustration and design by Sally Brown

DEDICATION

This book is simply, but with a great deal of love, dedicated to two individuals who have together shaped world thought in a way that benefits every individual living in it.

Edgar Cayce was born in 1877 in Hopkinsville, Kentucky, and lived a life that was sometimes painfully eventful. He had developed a gift in former lifetimes, however, which gave him the capacity to lie down and enter a state of altered consciousness that could then be tapped. He was able to touch in on the akashic records and the information in what we call universal consciousness.

He could contact the unconscious mind of individuals far distant from where he was giving a reading and could describe not only past lives, but also the state of the inquirer's physiological functioning and what needed to be done to return that individual to full health.

His legacy for the world was a library full of nearly 15,000 psychic readings of such depth that they have not been equalled in this century, if, indeed, in any century. Hundreds of books have been written about this man and his readings, and thousands upon thousands of men and women and particularly children have awakened to new life through the use of the information he left. I have not seen such a legacy rivaled in the thirty-seven years I have spent working with psychic data and this material as it related to the practice of medicine.

Edgar Cayce called his work the work of the Christ, and anyone who studies these readings to any depth would most likely agree. I certainly find it to be so.

I could not stop there. For, without the lifetime that Hugh Lynn Cayce (Edgar's eldest son) spent working with the readings, bringing the Work of the Christ to the attention of the world through his leadership, his traveling, speaking, writing, and enthusiasm, the A.R.E. would probably not now be in existence and the work of Edgar Cayce would lie in a dusty corner somewhere.

Too, this book and hundreds of others would not have been written. Nor would my life have been spent moving in the direction that Edgar and Hugh Lynn pointed out to all of us.

Hugh Lynn Cayce, like his father, has shaped thousands of lives with his love and his insights into the nature of humanity and what this world is all about. I would be deficient in my dedication if I did not place these two men together as world leaders in developing the understanding of why this world exists and what we are doing on it. Such an understanding is needed in the world today.

Edgar passed through God's Other Door in 1945 and Hugh Lynn in 1982. But I know that the future will point to these two men as examples of how the world can be changed by dedicating one's life to God's work. Thus, it is with a great deal of love and appreciation that I dedicate this book to Edgar and Hugh Lynn Cayce, who (if they could be heard) would want me to include the hundreds and hundreds of those who followed and made that work that much more important. And, Hugh Lynn, I hear you talking!

William A. McGarey, M.D.

TABLE OF CONTENTS

Foreword

There is no zealot like the nonbeliever who has seen the light. I suppose I fit that description when it comes to castor oil. As a child, I had too many distasteful encounters with a concoction my mother made by adding a liberal dose of castor oil to my orange juice and making sure that I forced it down. I hated the taste, and for years afterward avoided orange juice because of the unpleasant association.

Today, thanks to having been enlightened by Dr. William A. McGarey, I'm a true believer that we can enjoy the health benefits of "the oil that heals" without drinking a drop of it. Consequently, I keep a bottle of it close at hand and use it often. Castor oil often seems miraculous, for who would expect so many beneficial medicinal effects—everything from preventing abdominal surgery to dissolving gallstones and eliminating warts—from a common, inexpensive lubricant, used mostly today for industrial purposes.

In describing cases of magical recoveries by his patients

who applied castor oil, Dr. Bill reminds me of a New England doctor who years ago proclaimed the health benefits of drinking water laced with honey and vinegar. It is so simple and inexpensive, one wonders why all doctors don't recommend it.

But Dr. Bill does much more here than tell poignant success stories of sick people who got well by applying the oil he often recommends. He offers us a basic education about the healing process itself—a process misunderstood by those who believe that it is the doctor or the drug, or both, that heals us. Not so, says the author, based on his long experience as a family physician. Healing is a natural God-given function of the body, in collaboration with the mind and spirit. Disease or a failure to heal signals a dysfunction in one or all systems.

Dr. McGarey, a true medical pioneer, has shown great courage in betting his professional reputation on this concept, which he learned from studying and testing the concepts found in the Edgar Cayce readings, because it is very disturbing to many elements of the health care community. Many mainstream practitioners scoff at this "unscientific" theory—although it is one that is much more widely accepted today than when Dr. McGarey began practicing it over twenty years ago at the A.R.E. Clinic he founded in Phoenix, Arizona. Many patients reject this concept of healing because they would rather believe they are the victim of an external cause than take personal responsibility for their condition. And the "disease-care industry," as Dr. C. Norman Shealy describes the hospital-health insurance business, finds this concept threatening. It could reduce health problems if we learn to give our body-mind-spirit all the natural advantages needed to promote self-healing. Dr. Bill is doing his very best to teach us how.

While some health practitioners may regard "the oil that heals" as just another "snake oil" or placebo, readers will learn that Dr. McGarey's clinical research has demonstrated that the application of castor oil externally to the abdomen can increase significantly the total lymphocyte count, thus strengthening the body's immune system. The results of this preliminary testing at the A.R.E. Clinic, financed by a grant from the Fetzer Foundation, should be enough to justify much greater research into the healing mechanism triggered by castor oil.

Meanwhile, Dr. Bill continues to do what he feels called to do, a humble healer with a noble mission that is served well by this valuable book. It is a worthy addition to any library, as a primer for understanding the growing awareness of "energy medicine" and as a handy reference for when to use the oil for many minor ailments and serious dysfunctions. For as a country doctor he quotes once said, "Castor oil will leave the body in better condition than it found it."

That's a sound prescription for us all.

A. Robert Smith
Editor
Venture Inward magazine

Introduction

THERE REALLY ISN'T A MIRACLE CURE FOR ANYTHING, for miracles are just amazing happenings that come about from application of truths lodged somewhere in the realm of the yet-unexplained laws of the universe. However, it seems like a miracle when someone gently rubs a bit of castor oil over and over on a skin cancer of the ear, for instance, and the cancer just gradually disappears. It might take days or weeks or a few months, but it just doesn't make good sense. For who would attribute miraculous powers to a substance as lowly as castor oil? Yet this has happened, and the owner of the lesion on the ear feels as if he or she has discovered a new world. It's really a miracle to that individual.

This book is not about miracles, but it certainly has its foundation in the kind of healing that takes place when castor oil is used on—and sometimes in—the human body. Castor oil has a specific kind of an effect which some have called vibratory, when it is used therapeutically. For the present time, however, it probably is proper to say that the method of healing by using this oil is still undetermined. The results, however, have been apparent—not only in my experience, but in ancient times, as well as earlier in this century as reported in the medical literature.

It was twenty-six years ago that I first wrote a book about the use of castor oil in the practice of medicine. At that time, the manuscript was intended to be a simple report on the use of castor oil packs in the healing process of the human being. It was a monograph.

However, after the first couple of years, it became obvious that the book would be helpful for the lay reader in searching out ways of improving one's health and general welfare, in addition to alleviating the symptoms of an illness. So the monograph became a book. And it came to be called *Edgar Cayce and the Palma Christi.*

Now, after forty-six years in the practice of medicine and more than thirty-eight years as a student who has put into practice the concepts found in the Edgar Cayce readings, and after thousands of copies of the *Palma Christi* have found their way into the hands of the general public, I feel it is important to update and add to the original manuscript. I am including some of the more important lessons I've learned and some of the interesting happenings that have come my way as my patients, my family, and my friends have used the castor oil packs on their own bodies.

Also, as these years have passed by, I've found the Bible and its contents coming into close association with the human being and a person's amazing capabilities to become healed, and I've found the mind (the conscious and the subconscious) to be the link among the body, the emotions, and the spiritual essence of what we really are. The Bible with its wisdom, the Edgar Cayce readings, the mind, and the body are all interrelated through the use of these amazing castor oil packs, as you'll see as you follow my adventures through the pages of this book. It has truly been an amazing journey for me through this environment we call the earth plane.

My most vivid memory of one part of the Bible—the 23rd Psalm—has me standing with my portable tape recorder in the very center of the Greek theater located just a stone's throw from the spot where Aesculapius is said to have had his temple of sleeping and dreaming; where legend says that those who suffered with a diversity of illnesses came, slept, dreamed, and—in their sleep and dreaming—they were healed. I was standing there, surrounded by the ghosts of memories, listening to and recording the voice of Hugh Lynn Cayce, the son of Edgar Cayce, as he stood in the highest row of seats in this acoustically near-perfect theater, whispering the words of his favorite psalm.

The latter portion seems especially significant here: "Thou preparest a table before me in the presence of mine enemies: thou anointest my head with oil; my cup runneth over. Surely goodness and mercy shall follow me all the days of my life: and I will dwell in the house of the Lord for ever." (v. 5-6) Jesus was called the Christ, the Anointed One, for the Christ means "anointed." The mind of humanity through the centuries, apparently, has known that oil is necessary for anointing, though one cannot easily say why. One type of union with God, certainly, is symbolized by the anointing with oil. Is this perhaps a healing of another portion of ourselves?

To my mind, this is not unlikely for my experience has taught me that the greatest mystery in the universe is not outer space; it is not what might be found in the depths of the earth; but rather it is in the innermost parts of the human being, you or me, the entity, the soul that God created in the beginning and made in His image as a spiritual being.

These three seemingly diverse subjects—Aesculapius, the 23rd Psalm, and my chosen life profession—all appear to be related: dreaming is not only for the health of the mind, anointing is not only of the spirit, and healing is certainly not only of the physical body.

Perhaps it was, in part, this background which led me to begin investigation into the use of an oil which has its origins in antiquity; which, in turn, has almost been discarded by medical practice today; but which, in his psychic discourses for those who were ill, Edgar Cayce advocated for more than fifty different conditions of illness in the human body and to which he attributed some quite remarkable qualities.

Castor oil is still used in medicine as a cathartic, but my use of it in the form of a pack came about because of my familiarity with the Cayce readings, because of my study of them, and because I saw literally hundreds of instances in which such packs were advised for conditions of the body that seemed to be—in most instances—unrelated to each other. Yet each person was advised to use the same therapy.

It would be difficult to state now for what kind of condition I first recommended the use of the castor oil pack. As results came, however, its utilization became more and more frequent. After three or four years, I began my earlier report, which eventually became the book dealing with my experiences up to that time.

In the years that have passed since that first attempt to record the changes that occur within the physiological functioning of the body from the use of castor oil, literally thousands of individuals have benefited by castor oil applied as a pack and as a substance to be rubbed onto the body. There is probably no portion of the external human anatomy that has not been treated with this remarkable substance.

Then why not call it "the oil that heals"?

Part I

Chapter One

Don't Forget to Smell the Dandelions

WHEN I WAS A FIVE-YEAR-OLD BOY playing on the hills that rimmed the Ohio valley, I discovered a magnificent flower. It had a wonderful yellow-orange face to it, which magically changed after a few weeks to a fluffy white ball of what my parents called seeds. To me, they were one of nature's miracles—I could pick one of those long-stemmed objects of wonderment, hold it close to my mouth and gently blow, and off they would go, these little white floaters, into the wind to land far away from my sight.

But the flower itself carried even more interest for me. I used to lie down on the grass and smell the dandelion as it was clothed in all its glory. I wondered about that bit of nature. My nose told me there was not much of an odor, but an aroma of some sort did seem to be there. And I wondered, "What can the dandelion be good for?"

In my later years, it occurred to me that perhaps memories of a past life as a doctor using herbs could have been

1

stirred deep within me, to give me that early interest in the dandelion. Most people think it is simply a weed, especially when it gets a good start on one's lawn.

But that memory of lying there on the grass, not far from my home, smelling the dandelion has made its place in my life ever since. It symbolized for me the inquisitive spirit that must be in all individuals, if they are to understand their origin, their destiny, and the nature of all those mysteries that are locked within every created object that becomes part of our personal experience.

The dandelion (*Taraxacum officinale*), as a matter of fact, is a highly respected herb, nutritious in its nature and used to clear obstructions from and to stimulate the liver to detoxify poisons in the system. It has a strong alkalinizing effect to neutralize acids and acts as an eliminatory herb in maintaining body health and as a building agent. The leaves and the root are the active ingredients most commonly used, and dandelion tea is applied most frequently in renal, bladder, and liver difficulties.[1]

Perhaps the flower is there to catch one's attention and thrill all those who are, by nature, inquisitive and investigative. But there is a value, too, and I've found that most of nature—given us through the kindness of God—is here to be used for aid and for help, once its use is determined.

The experience with the dandelion has proved to me that the commonplace things one tends to neglect in travels through the earth are often uncommon in their true value, so let's always remember—even when we are grown and relatively sophisticated—to smell the dandelions.

It was not long after that that my mother died following surgery for pulmonary tuberculosis. I was seven, and I—like my two brothers—cried when I found out that mother had left us and would not be seen again. Some years later, when the idea of reincarnation became part of my belief system, I understood death as a passage from one room to another, from one environment which we call the earth plane to a spiritual setting where the surroundings are of a different vibratory nature. When we make that change, it is really I or you who steps into that other dimension.

When my mother died, I wasn't wise enough to smell the dandelions in that experience. Looking back, however, I know there is truth in the concept that every experience is an opportunity for soul growth. If life is indeed continuous, my inner being must have been aware of that reality, and what Edgar Cayce had to say about it was my inner lesson:

> *Life is continuous! The soul moves on,* gaining by each experience that necessary for its comprehending of its kinship and relationship to Divine. (1004-2)

My belief system was rooted early in the Presbyterian church, although I have had past incarnations, too, as a Catholic priest. But in this life, I chose parents who had adopted the Presbyterian approach to their understanding of the Divine. From the time I was twelve years old, I taught others about the biblical story. At first, I taught seven- and eight-year-old students. After many years, I taught adults. In between, I aimed my life toward the ministry, but changed it midstream to medical education.

But my faith included the view of a Creative Force in the universe—and even outside the universe—which brought me into being and which created all things. This view brought me later to the writings of the Chinese mystic, Lao Tsu. He found the Divine to be the Mother of the Ten Thousand Things, and just as much of a mystery. These few words, however, from the *Tao Te Ching*[2] helped me feel more in touch with that which I could not truly explain:

> Something, in veiled creation, came to be
> Before the earth was formed, or heaven.

In the silence, apart, alone,
It changes not, is ever present, never failing—
Think of it as the Mother of the Ten Thousand Things.

It seems to me now that we need a basis from which to
start understanding the mystery of the body and that which
brought it into being. I didn't look at life in exactly that way
during my formative years, but what was happening inside
my unconscious mind was the adoption of the idea of God
as the Creative Force, the Beginning of all things, the Wisdom that created me with His potential and made the path
clear for the return voyage. And I accepted Jesus as the
Christ, the Anointed One, who had already made the trip
back to His beginning and who had performed something
mystical here in the Earth that is still difficult to understand.
Another experience for me, another step.

Communication has always been important to me. When I
was in the eighth grade, my teacher told me I would some
day write a book—she apparently saw that in my writing.
From the time I was eleven years old until I finished college,
I worked in some capacity with newspapers. Paperboy,
printer's devil (they had those in the '30s), reporter, typeset-
ter, printer, and—for a period of several months when the
editor of the small-town newspaper was down with a heart
attack—I was the acting editor of the paper—at age eighteen.

In college I took part in writing, helping to create a liter-
ary publication, writing poetry and short stories, and
helping with the college newspaper, editing it in my final
year. It seemed that writing was something that had to be
part of my destiny, wherever I found myself. The experiences that came about during those years taught me how to
communicate, but one cannot communicate unilaterally.
To write a story for the newspaper, I had to ask questions
and listen to those who knew what was happening. Then
I put my talents to work.

It must be that way, to some extent, as we work with our physical body. If we pay no attention to what our body is telling us, we may end up with a perforated ulcer of the stomach instead of the earlier overacidity. Listening will tell us that something is wrong, something is burning in our stomach. Why not listen and give the communication a response—change our diet, our life style a bit, and introduce some antacid preparation?

One of the most frequent criticisms I hear about today's physicians is that they don't listen. Patients tell me this, their voices ringing with resentment and anger, for they all believe they know something about their own body. It is, after all, their body. They know how they feel. And to them, how they feel is important. If their doctor won't listen, frustration results and there is further disruption of the physical body because of the emotional upheaval.

Communication is always a two-way street. Knowledge of our body requires a sensitivity to what is going on and a response to that need. It doesn't always take a doctor to know when something is happening inside, and then what our conscious response brings about in the way of correction.

Sometimes, like a rumor that a reporter catches on the fly, there is a hint of something going wrong inside the body that comes in an instructive dream. Both the rumor and the dream need investigation. Once investigated and interpreted, the rumor may become fact that can be published in the paper and the dream may become a therapy that can be instituted in the body. The key is to listen, appraise, then act.

Chapter Two
Medical School and Early Practice Years

EXPERTS ABOUND IN ALL MEDICAL SCHOOLS, AND MY classmates saw them as the fountainhead of all knowledge—gurus, in a sense. Much knowledge, but little philosophy. Philosophers are rare indeed in medical halls of learning. They are present, but their voices are outnumbered, unheard, or discounted. Existence of a Higher Power, a Creative Energy, a God, was not acknowledged in my four years of medical schooling. Except, perhaps, in the form of profanity.

I recall clearly a particularly wild argument I had with John Miley, one of my classmates. He was saying, "That's what the experts say in the textbooks." I was telling him why their statements did not make sense to me, and questioning why I should accept their point of view. Common sense—philosophy—does not often find its way into medical literature.

Early in my practice of medicine, a pathologist was looking at a section of the appendix which had been removed. He told me it showed appendicitis. I looked at the specimen and asked the doctor how many lymphocytes had to be there to designate it as appendicitis instead of a normal appendix. He shrugged off the question, but I persisted because normally the appendix does have lymphocytes present when nothing is wrong. Such a presence is, in fact, a part of the immune system, which encompasses all the lymphatic tissue in the body. It appeared to me that the number of lymphocytes present simply gave the pathologist an opportunity to make an educated guess. His guess was "appendicitis." My pathologist was unhappy with me, but he didn't know that I used to smell dandelions.

I found out from these two experiences that all things are not really as they seem. The experts are not always right, as we often assume, and disease is not an on/off phenomenon, but rather a process found active within the physiology of the human body.

Medical school did teach me, however, about the structure of the body, about physiology, something about the various specialties, a great deal about pharmacology, much about pathology—the end point of a disease process—but most significantly we were taught about diseases, how to recognize them when they appear (sometimes as if by magic), and how to do battle with them. We were not taught that the body frequently has amazing abilities to overcome the beginning stages of a disease process, if given a bit of help here and there. And we were not given any instruction about nutrition, dietary practices, or the effect of these upon the health of the body. Nor were emotions and their direct effect upon the functioning of the body given credence.

I was impressed by the work which Richard Vilter, one of my professors, had done in the field of vitamins, and I could not understand why the use of vitamins as an aid to the body was not more widespread. I tested vitamins early in my medical school career, and I found that I had more energy and simply felt better when I used them. Another insight—something good might be happening within the body tissues when you simply feel better. But arguments still rage about what vitamins do and do not accomplish.

A good night's sleep will often make one feel better. Seeing someone you love will do the same. A good hug—or a bunch of hugs—will enhance that same feeling. Recent work has shown that one feels worse when one frowns, feels better if one puts a smile on one's face—no matter how "down" the person may feel prior to the smile. And, if things get worse, laugh! That's another way to move toward happier, feeling-better times. To a degree, those happier times spell healing of the body.

It was shortly after I began my practice of medicine in my home town of Wellsville, Ohio, that I discovered another way to gain an insight into myself—another way to smell the dandelions. It was a very busy time, and house calls were still a way of life in that mid-Western town.

After an especially busy day including house calls, surgery in the morning, and a full day at the office, I finally climbed into bed. When the phone rang shortly after midnight, I groaned. I was summoned on another call, and I grumbled all the way to my car, vowing to charge five dollars instead of the usual three.

When I returned home, more like a pussy cat than the roaring lion, I tried to sneak into bed without waking my wife. But she heard me and said, "Well, did you charge them like you said you would?" I told her I didn't—that the little girl was really sick, and besides, they didn't have any money to pay me for the visit. We went to sleep again.

It was at that point that I became aware that service was what I was there for and I chose it. My later years emphasized that concept of service and enlarged on it, for how is the quality of Divine Love best manifested, unless it is in helping those who need help, caring for those who are anxious and insecure, those who are sick in body, mind, or spirit?

Chapter Three
A Chance Encounter

(If Chance Is Yet a Reality)

NOTHING REALLY HAPPENS BY CHANCE, DOES IT? AT least that was what I was to find repeated over and over again in the Edgar Cayce readings. I was now in the practice of medicine in Phoenix, Arizona, having started over again after a stint in the air force as a flight surgeon.

It was 1955, and I had been in town just a few months. I had started an exploratory adventure into the field of parapsychology with a friend of mine, Dr. Bill Rogers. We had come across a wonderful story about Edgar Cayce—a man who could lie down on a couch and enter an altered state of consciousness—and really tell what was happening inside the body of another individual who could be 2,000 miles away. It was as if he were communicating with the unconscious mind of another person, while his own conscious mind was set aside. I was fascinated, but thought—"Well, that's just another event in the past, for Cayce died in 1945."

Then, one day, my receptionist came rushing into the office and gave me the phone number of a man who was going to talk about Edgar Cayce. It was Cayce's oldest son, Hugh Lynn Cayce, and I was excited.

That was the beginning of the adventure that was to take me through time and space, in a sense, and demand my time and attention, my thought processes, and my writing and speaking abilities for the rest of my life. For there is still much to be done, some thirty-eight years after that "chance encounter." It was Hugh Lynn Cayce who captured my imagination that day after I made the phone call. And the world was a different place from that point onward.

Hugh Lynn told about his father's abilities that night at a lecture, and I began to understand how this psychic information could relate to the practice of medicine. Much of Edgar Cayce's life was spent in giving 14,306 "readings," as they came to be called. Over a period of forty years, two-thirds of these readings—9,604—were given for individuals who were ill; some seriously so. The remainder were for a variety of other reasons. The bulk of his work, then, had to do with what I've been trained in and involved with for most of my life—the care of those who are ill.

The full story of his life is well told by Thomas Sugrue in his book *There Is a River*,[3] which is biographical in nature. Later on, Jess Stearn authored a best seller about Cayce, *The Sleeping Prophet*,[4] which emphasizes more the importance of Cayce's physical readings. Since then, literally hundreds of books have been published about this man or his work, which he stated was the work of the Christ.

Cayce died in 1945, but while he lived he was able to lie down on a couch or bed, loosen his tie and collar, and place his folded hands on his forehead. After a few moments, he would bring his hands down over his solar plexus, and enter a state that resembled trance or self-hypnosis. It has been called in recent years an altered state of consciousness.

In this state, he was able, upon suggestion by the conductor of the reading, to visualize, describe, and comment upon another individual who might be thousands of miles distant at that moment and a complete stranger to Cayce and those surrounding him. He was able to describe physical conditions which were present in that person's body, in the bloodstream, the nervous system, or other parts of the person's physiology; and then give suggestions, which, if followed, tended to restore that body back to a more normal condition of health. Each time Cayce "went to sleep" and gave such information for an individual, this, with the questions and answers, became a reading.[5]

Cayce's clairvoyance, while in this condition, was substantiated time and again, and he subsequently became known nationally as The Miracle Man of Virginia Beach, Virginia,[6] where he spent his last years. His abilities to be accurate in the unconscious state throughout his life brought a variety of people to see him and ask him questions. During the days of World War II, the mail brought literally thousands of letters pleading for help for servicemen who were embroiled in the war and had not been heard from. He was indeed an unusual man who apparently had direct contact with a source of information few people have had in recorded history.

Cayce's strength—in this field of parapsychology—was his medical clairvoyance. He described the body differently than anyone else I had ever met or read about. Certainly he did not discuss it in the way I had been taught in my medical school training. He talked about "forces" in the body—meaning the energy in the bloodstream or the nervous system—the digestive activities, and all those activities that go on within the body. He talked about incoordination, about "overflow of nerve impulses," about lacteal ducts, about the Peyer's patches in the small intestine. It was a new education in how to help the body to become healed and to return to a normal balance.

It took me quite a while to look at this wonderful human body from a perspective different from what I had been taught.

One of the earliest readings in which castor oil packs were suggested by Cayce was for a woman who had applied for a reading because of a tumor of the upper bowel—diagnosed by x-ray as cancer, but stated in the reading to be an impaction. This reading was taken on August 17, 1927, and represented the beginning of a type of therapy which was continued throughout the life of this psychic individual, who, without a medical training or degree, found himself in the position of diagnosing illnesses and giving suggestions for therapy, without seeing the patient or often even knowing anything about the person, except the location of the individual.

In another reading (1836-1) Cayce described what he saw in the functioning of a sixty-two-year-old man who had epilepsy and advised what to do:

As we find, unless there are measures taken the conditions here may become very serious.

These are the conditions as we find them with this body, [1836]:

There having been a disturbance in the lacteal ducts, there has been a disturbance that causes an adhesion in this portion of the body; and at times a drawing in the side (right) just below the liver and gall duct area.

This disassociation causes a breakage in the coordinating of the cerebrospinal and sympathetic nervous system, until there are the tendencies and impulses for an overflow of the nerve impulse through the cerebrospinal system.

And these, unless some measures are taken, may

form a clot or a break on the brain.

As to the general conditions of the body, these are gradually giving away to these disturbances, both from the physical reaction and from the anxiety in the self as well as those about the body.

Then, as we find:

We would apply, consistently, for at least ten such applications, the castor oil packs—about every other evening, when the body is ready to retire, for an hour; the packs changed about twice during the hour period. These would be applied over the caecum and the gall duct area, or the right side from the ribs to the point of the hip, extending lower over the abdomen in that area, see? Use about three thicknesses of flannel, wrung out of the hot castor oil and applied, then a pad put over same, and then the electric pad or dry heat put over same to keep it warm or as hot as the body can stand it, see? Do this every other evening for at least *ten* such applications, making a period of twenty days, see?

Also, *each* evening, for at least twenty to thirty days, we would massage the spine—downward; beginning at the base of the brain; one day using *olive oil,* the next day using cocoa butter. Massage all the body will absorb. Let this extend on either side of the spinal column, from the base of the brain to the end of the spine; gently, in a rotary motion, massaged into the body, see? Rub *away from* the head, always. Take about twenty to thirty minutes each evening to give this massage, see?

After the massage, as *also* after the castor oil packs, the body may be sponged off—the areas of the massage *and* the packs—with lukewarm soda water if desired.

In the diet—keep away from fried foods and from

any hog meat of *any* kind—especially sausage or the like. (1836-1)

Cayce went on to assure the man that if he were to follow the directions, he would find assistance in eliminating the disturbance in his body.

Chapter Four
Healing as an Awakening in Consciousness

EDGAR CAYCE, IN THE YEARS PRIOR TO HIS death in 1945, seemed to have an affinity for castor oil. In most quarters, though, it has been held with disdain, since its action on the intestinal tract, when taken in large doses by mouth, is sometimes explosive. Nevertheless, Cayce advocated it hundreds of times in his readings, offering the oil as an aid in bringing the body back to a state of normalcy. Most often, however, it was to be applied on the body, not in it.

One inquirer, seeking help for himself from the sleeping Cayce, asked if he should take the oil by mouth. The reply was that if you have a castor oil consciousness, take castor oil. This was a revelation to me. I was just beginning to understand that Cayce, from his unconscious mind, was dealing with illnesses from a perspective that I had not yet encountered. And it began to make sense. Cayce was approaching things from the standpoint of consciousness and need. What does that mean in a practical sense?

When I first started reading the Cayce material, a patient came to see me who was very definitive in his approach to remedies. He had a sore throat and he told me that penicillin always took care of his sore throats and that's what he wanted. Before reading Cayce's statement about consciousness and castor oil, I would have been a bit dismayed by the man's wanting penicillin. However, the idea of consciousness gave me new insights. Perhaps this man had a penicillin consciousness! If so, he would respond to it. And he did.

What does penicillin consciousness mean? Perhaps it is better understood as a manifestation of faith. Why, for instance, am I a Presbyterian? I was born into the faith (by choice, of course, if we truly have that power before being born), and I believed the tenets I learned in the church. So I naturally would respond, in my spiritual development, to the ideas in that church more readily than in the Baptist, for instance, or Greek Orthodox, or whatever. I had a Presbyterian consciousness.

The incident with the penicillin, along with Cayce's statement, made it a lot easier for me to understand that everyone has a different approach, a different road to travel as he or she moves through an incarnation. And I needed to be sensitive about what would help patients most—as nearly as I could tell—in their search for healing. If they have a castor oil consciousness, they get castor oil. If they have a surgical consciousness, they undoubtedly need surgery. Or manipulation or radiation or chemotherapy. People need what they truly need until they change their own consciousness in a manner that manifests a different need.

As this bit of information sank into my awareness sufficiently to put it into action, I also became aware of another pertinent factor in the healing process: there is an awakening of consciousness—a psychic event—within the tissues of the body whenever true healing comes about. And the therapy that is used carries within it an essence, a power that enables that awakening to come about. Perhaps it is the faith mentioned earlier that is the pathway, but the power is the creative element that stimulates the atoms and cells into a new awareness. Cayce described it like this:

> For, all healing comes from the one source. And whether there is the application of foods, exercise, medicine, or even the knife—it is to bring [to] the consciousness of the forces within the body that aid in reproducing themselves—the awareness of creative or God forces. (2696-1)

It has been vitally interesting for me to probe into the unconscious images Cayce presented about what we are as human beings. The "forces," for instance. All tissue is composed of atoms, and it was Cayce's point of view that all atoms have consciousness. Consciousness is a "force" when applied in any situation. Thus Cayce termed those aggregations of atoms and cells as "forces." And they, knowing their origin after having been awakened by the Divine, respond by attaining their normal status. Some people call this healing, or a cure.

Castor oil packs became the first Cayce therapy I applied in my practice of medicine. It had been described so often in the readings and seemed so simple to use and so innocuous. The results seemed remarkable to me and to the patient. How could an oil pack, applied with a heating pad, bring about the resolution of an intestinal problem or an abscess of the axilla? Or a gallbladder attack? Or a phlebitis of the leg? But these things did happen, and I was compelled to look deeper.

Chapter Five
Castor Oil as a Healing Force

I HAVE ALWAYS BELIEVED THAT WE CAN TELL more about the truth of what is happening inside the human body by studying the individual who is ill rather than consulting a set of data and getting lost in statistics. Dr. Richard Lee wrote about this concept.[7] He pointed out that observations of single events in medicine, published or unpublished, are today "condescendingly called anecdotes; stories concocted by well-meaning but scientifically naive clinicians."

Dr. Lee suggests that numbers and statistics have taken the place of the careful attention to the individual case and the commonplace, previously in the field of medicine recognized as the hallmark of the excellent clinician. He asks, "How many important and interesting biologic events go unnoticed by blinkered academicians working single-mindedly at collecting series of patients or diseases being enough to publish?"

In his paper, Lee reminds us that modern medicine, along with the culture that has shaped it, has noted a steady decline in appreciation and respect for the individual and the unique. "One test, one patient, one problem cannot begin to satisfy the voracious appetite statistically significant doctors have for multitudes of numbers and crowds of patients... For the best possible outcome, each patient needs, and has a right to expect, his/her doctor's undivided attention and effort. To judge the patient, the illness, and the medical effort only by averages and percentages demeans both patient and doctor and diminishes the importance of illness ... "

Some of the most important discoveries in medicine have been through observation of only one patient. And Dr. Lee's message is to keep on seeing the value in single observations. I would add that we need to keep on discovering the mysteries that lie within that human being who has unfortunately fallen ill.

Illness has a purpose and I'm sure it is one associated with learning at the deepest level of the human being. The soul undergoing the experience knows this fact. There is an eternal need for greater understanding of oneself that can come about only from the learning experiences given each person and met in a constructive, helpful manner. These awarenesses always move one forward toward fulfillment of the greater purpose in life. Cayce talked about what one's purpose might be:

> The purpose in life, then, is not the gratifying of appetites nor of any selfish desires, but it is that the entity, the soul, may make the earth ... a better place in which to live. (4047-2)

The goal and the purpose were a bit different, Cayce often indicated. The goal, he said, was to come to the point of knowing ourselves to be ourselves, yet one with God, or the Creative Forces. That brings the goal and the purpose, the heavens and the earth, closer together in our understanding.

To put Dr. Lee's words into action, let's look at a number of single events, and see if they do not spark a new awareness in our minds. The people involved in the following events found the value in castor oil as they explored its use for conditions that afflicted their own bodies.

CASTOR OIL FOR HERNIAS

Healing of the human body comes about in a variety of ways, but the Cayce readings emphasize the concept that consciousness of the individual is the real determining factor. Every organ, every cell, every atom has its own type of consciousness. Each part of God's world, down to its molecular and atomic structure, is aware of its own individual job, its origin and its destiny, as a manifestation of the Creative Forces of the universe.

This is one of the reasons why I am fascinated by the variety of illnesses and conditions of the body that respond to the oil of the lowly castor bean. It can certainly cleanse the body—most of us recall that effect clearly from our childhood, when we are given a bit of that oil to clean us out. If cleansing is part of the nature of consciousness of castor oil, then logically it will cleanse wherever it is applied. Proper cleansing allows cellular structures to function more normally and often to regenerate themselves.

A recent letter reminded me of this. It came from a man who had suffered a condition usually cleared up only by surgery—inguinal hernia. When he was seventy-one, he began wearing a standard hernia support because he felt a strain in the left inguinal area. Four years later the same condition showed up on the right side, so he switched to a double hernia support. Later on that year, when his right hernia bulged out rather severely, he underwent surgery on that side.

For the next two years he continued wearing the appliance on the left side, but neither side "felt real good." So, he started to massage both areas with hot castor oil, using a rotary motion—clockwise on the left, counterclockwise on the right.

"I did this in units of 100 massage strokes, then rested for a while and repeated ten or twelve more units," he told me. "Consequently, each area received 1,000 to 1,200 rotary strokes. Castor oil was applied liberally during the massage and perhaps two to three tablespoonfuls were absorbed by the body. When finished, I would not wash but just wiped off the surplus oil with paper towels. In several weeks both areas felt better. I followed the massage procedure three or four times a week. In several months, things were greatly improved."

He no longer wore a hernia belt, only an athletic supporter. Occasionally he noticed discomfort and some swelling, but those conditions cleared up after several months. He continued the massages once or twice a week as insurance. When he wrote, at age seventy-nine and a year-and-a-half after starting the oil treatments, he reported that his condition had cleared up: "I lift whatever has to be lifted. Once it was necessary to lift 100 pounds. In fact, I don't think about the hernia any more."

I agree with my correspondent when he tells me, "I'm sure the massage was a factor in my healing. However, I strongly feel the castor oil that was absorbed by my body did a great deal of good."

Such an experience is exhilarating—to him and to me. This patient's experience is much like Cayce's comments on how healing comes about:

Know that all strength, all healing of every nature is the changing of the vibrations from within—the attuning of the Divine within the living tissue of a body to Creative Energies. This alone is healing. Whether it is accomplished by the use of drugs, the knife or whatnot, it is the attuning of the atomic structure of the living cellular force to its spiritual heritage. (1967-1)

Keep this awareness within your own inner being and you'll experience a leap in consciousness every time you overcome an illness of the physical body.

CHRONIC PROBLEMS

In understanding the body, I think it is important to recognize that every portion of the body tends to maintain a status quo. Very few people really like change, and change must take place if healing is to occur or if the patient is going to progress in consciousness. Purveyors of change usually are not welcome. If they are in the form of therapies of any kind, the total body consciousness will often rebel and prevent positive results.

It's somewhat like a computer. When the computer is programmed in a certain manner, hitting the proper sequence of keys will always give the same readout. It's difficult to change the programming, and such change takes time.

The human body responds in a similar way. The castor oil pack might be compared to a new program as, over time, it affects the cells of the body and thus a new program is in operation.

Velma is a seventy-two-year-old woman who had a hysterectomy in 1965. The surgery seemed to have been all right, but since the operation—for the past twenty-three years—she has experienced constant gaseous distention, constipation, abdominal "miseries," edema of the ankles, and episodes where her gut would feel as if it were twisting in on itself. These periods would sometimes last for hours.

After being seen as a patient in our office, she was instructed on how to use a castor oil pack. She was faithful in following instructions and came back for a recheck in just two weeks.

She told us that within minutes after the very first pack was placed on her abdomen, she felt as though the gut inside the belly wall untwisted on itself. Since that time, there has been absolutely no recurrence of symptoms. She has no twisting sensations, her ankles are no longer edematous, and her abdominal "miseries," constipation, and gaseous distention are gone.

Some individuals are undoubtedly more sensitive than others. I've observed those who are severely reactive to smoke, while others are not. Some cannot take medicines, only herbal preparations. There are those individuals who cannot eat meat. Sensitivity also extends to those who tune in to their unconscious more than others.

This woman must have been one of those who are sensitive to the healing powers of castor oil. For she reported to us—and this is the most unusual aspect of her story—that since she's been using the packs, she has actually seen oil in her stools. And she's taken no oil by mouth.

It is interesting to consider what mechanisms might have taken part in restoring normalcy to someone like this elderly woman who has been bothered with a problem that has no known diagnosis, no obvious findings to the searching hands of a physician. Yet, for twenty-three years something was out of sync, something that was incoordinant inside her body. And the vibration or effect of the castor oil brought about a normal function once again.

Another longstanding problem had its origin in 1964, when Richard Disney was injured playing football. He had a back operation the next year and again in 1980, the latter to remove part of a crushed disc.

In 1987, he reinjured the area. Following some chiropractic adjustments, he was able to go back to work after just a few days. Several weeks later, however, he developed sciatic pain on his left side and had several more treatments from the chiropractor. The treatments were combined with bed rest, electrical stimulation, Motrin®, aspirin, Tylenol®, ice, heat, and massage. He had "the works" in terms of normal therapy; but instead of improving, all the symptoms worsened.

He had been a member of the A.R.E. for a number of years and was reading some of the material I had written about castor oil packs on the day that he had actually given up and had been seen by his family doctor. He reports: "The doctor set up an appointment for me with a neurosurgeon for the next day. That evening, Ellen [his wife] applied a castor oil pack for one hour to my lower back. I felt some relief afterward, but was still in a lot of pain.

"At this point, I was convinced that surgery was the only course of action left. The surgeon examined me, set up a myelogram, blood tests, and x-rays for the next week. My wife continued applying castor oil packs and heat daily.

"After seven days of the packs and a few doses of olive oil, the pain was completely gone. I canceled all appointments. After a two-day break, my wife Ellen applied the castor oil packs daily for another three days. I have not had any recurrence of back or sciatic pain. We also used the same kind of packs on a cyst that my wife had on her leg. It started to drain after three applications and has caused her no more problems.

"I am convinced that I have experienced a miracle and I am thankful to my Higher Power, my wife's persistence and faith, and the information provided in your book at just the right time."

I also am glad that Richard experienced his miracle. I

understand better now why I had such a variety of experiences earlier in my life because they aided me in writing and communicating through articles and books so that I could be helpful to others, while at the same time aiding me in my own awakening process.

And what is the awakening process if not the soul growth that comes by using every experience in life creatively and constructively.

HOW DO YOU MAKE A CASTOR OIL PACK AND WHAT DOES IT DO?

To make a castor oil pack, you will need the following materials:

1. Flannel cloth
2. Plastic sheet—no coloring
3. Electric heating pad
5. Two or three safety pins
6. Castor oil
7. Bath towel

Prepare a soft flannel cloth, preferably of wool flannel. The cloth should be two or four thicknesses when folded, and should measure about ten by twelve or fourteen inches in size after being folded. This is the size needed for abdominal application. Other areas of the body would need to have the pack shaped and sized to the area to be treated.

Next, pour some castor oil onto the cloth, using a plastic sheet underneath to keep from soiling other articles. Make sure the cloth is wet but not dripping with oil. Apply the pack to the portion of the body that needs treatment, keeping the plastic sheet on the outside.

After that, place the heating pad on the plastic sheet, covering the pack, and turn the heat to low first, then to medium and higher if the body is comfortable with it. Do not burn the skin. This is not therapeutic!

Finally, wrap a bath towel, folded lengthwise, around the trunk of the person being treated, so that it covers the pack and the heating pad, and fasten it in place with safety pins.

The pack should remain in place for an hour to an hour and a half, and the skin can be easily cleansed with a solution of baking soda and water—two teaspoons to a quart. Use it warm, not cold.

The flannel pack need not be discarded after a single application, but may be kept in a plastic container for future use. Unless the pack gets discolored or the oil becomes rancid, it may continue to be used over a period of months. Some like to keep the pack in the refrigerator, but it should then always be warmed up before application.

Frequency of use? From three to seven days a week, to be followed most often after three treatments by olive oil (up to two teaspoonfuls is used most commonly), to stimulate the liver in its activity. Take a teaspoonful or more. Be careful about taking larger amounts.

The most obvious effect that I found in treating the body using a castor oil pack was the enhancement of the immune system. As a portion of their duties, the lymphatics—part of the immune system—drain all parts of the body. When the tissues in any area of the body are cleansed by the eliminatory process, the cells are in much better condition to work normally—and the activity of the immune bodies and substances are able better to do their job in defending the body or rebuilding it.

This has been my way of looking at these things. No proof, of course, but lots of patients are indeed happier than they were and in better health.

Although experiences like the foregoing do not get published in the literature because they seem so strange, the use of castor oil packs has proliferated over the years in many parts of the world and with many physicians and health care practitioners.

At one of our earlier medical symposia in Phoenix, a young orthopedic surgeon reported on how he had every bed on his floor equipped with a K-pack (a special heating pad) and a castor oil pack, and he used them routinely in postoperative situations. Other doctors in his hospital became interested and started using them, but the orthopod never told them that the packs were first described by a psychic. That would have lost his case right there!

Not too long ago, a story came to our attention at the A.R.E. Clinic here in Phoenix about a postoperative patient who nearly died. A licensed practical nurse told us the story; the patient was one to whom she was assigned in her hospital in the northwest part of our country.

The patient was delivered of her pregnancy by Caesarian section and was doing well with her baby, who also was thriving. On the third post-partum day, however, the mother started having trouble with her abdomen and the surgeons on the case agreed it was probably an intestinal obstruction. Surgery was recommended and performed, but the results were not as expected, and the patient's condition worsened. More surgery was not advised by the surgical team, and the mother's condition appeared to be deteriorating.

When the female obstetrician was searching for some helpful alternative, the nurse suggested to the doctor that she knew something about castor oil packs and that they might be helpful.

The packs were applied, and after fifteen hours the patient started to pass liquid stools, followed shortly by a normal bowel movement—and the crisis ended. Afterward, nothing was discussed about the packs, but I would suppose there was some awakening in the mind of that physician who was creative and open-minded enough to take a suggestion from a nurse about an unusual therapy, no matter how highly regarded the nurse may have been.

One of the powerful factors operating in the Edgar Cayce material is mystery. Cayce said that mystery excites the imagination of those who find it in their lives—and those who are ready to be awakened are stimulated and move to a greater awareness and a higher consciousness.

An unusual experience I had with serious illness and castor oil packs also involved intestinal obstruction. I was called to see an elderly woman at home; she was a longtime patient and unable to come to the office. She had developed a distended abdomen which worsened rapidly. She had lost her sense of humor, had quit watching her television programs, and had gone to bed.

When I examined her, I found that with her abdomen so grossly distended, the cause was obviously an obstruction and she needed to be hospitalized. A gastric tube had to be inserted in an effort to deflate the belly. She adamantly refused. She was well over eighty years of age, said that she was not going to leave her home and that if she was going to die, it was right there that she wanted to do it.

To ease her pain and discomfort, I instructed her daughter to place a castor oil pack on the abdomen without heat, but to keep it in place constantly. And the patient was to take ice chips to keep her hydrated.

The following day, she was feeling better and her abdomen was not quite as distended. Also, she had started to smile and joke once again. The next day she started having a few liquid stools and her distention was nearly gone. I gave her a suppository and she had a large, nearly normal bowel movement. The obvious diagnosis was a severe intestinal obstruction caused by a fecal impaction.

When I visited her on the third day, she was up in a chair, watching her favorite television programs. All systems were working and she had delayed her time of departure from this plane.

How did the castor oil pack act to make such a radical

change in direction in this woman's state of health? I would say that she had, prior to her illness, established a degree of homeostasis—a state of stability in her internal physiological environment, which for her spelled health.

Then something happened—probably having to do with her nutrition, which caused the fecal impaction to take place. That much we can understand. But when she worsened, what was it about the oil that loosened up the impaction and turned things around? Did the castor oil soak through to the intestinal tract? Was it a vibratory activity in the castor oil, after soaking through, or did it work as vibration without soaking through?

Because of the nature of this dimension in which all of us reside, we know that everything is in vibration. All substances in this physical environment are composed of atoms or subatomic particles. These are in constant motion and are one form of energy. All substances, then, whether they be living or not, give off vibrations which, given time and more research, will eventually be measured and shown to be uniquely specific in their own nature. Thus, castor oil will have a different vibratory force than peanut oil, for instance.

Is it really vibration, then, that carries the healing nature of the castor oil into the body to launch a new approach, a new situation, a new balance inside the structure and functioning of the body so that healing does, in fact, come about? Whatever brought about the change, by the time three days had passed the woman octogenarian had regained her sense of humor, was chatting with her daughter again, and was watching her television. And she was eating normally again. She had regained that state of homeostasis that, for her, added up to health.

It might be illustrated, like most events which occur in this dimension, on a graph showing happenings in time. (See Figure 1.)

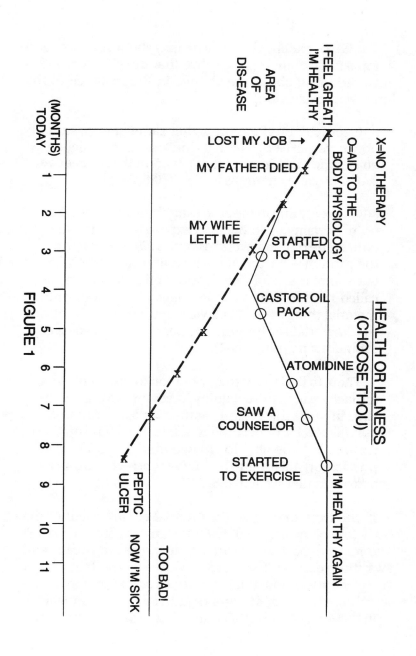

FIGURE 1

The Cayce readings had much to say about vibration, and it appears from their perspective that the vibratory influence did bring about the change in the instance of the intestinal obstruction:

Electricity or vibration is that same energy, same power, ye call God. Not that God is an electric light or an electric machine, but that vibration that is creative is of that same energy as life itself. (2828-4)

... everything in motion, everything that has taken on materiality as to become expressive in any kingdom in the material world, is *by* the *vibrations* that are the motions—or those positive and negative influences that make for that differentiation that man has called matter in its various stages of evolution into material things. For ... all vibration must eventually, as it materializes into matter, pass though a stage of evolution and out. (699-1)

Then, to find the correct vibration for elements that are lacking in their sustaining forces for a living organism, in such a way and manner as for same to be assimilated by, or become effective in, a living organism ... is to be able to change that environ of that physical organism as to be creative and evoluting in its activity in that system. (5576-1)

If one were to change the internal environment of the body (the physiology) so that it became creative, wouldn't one really expect a movement, then, toward health and away from disease? The mystery of the body certainly is not yet fully understood, but it continues to be exciting as one searches, as one stops long enough to smell the dandelions.

In our work at the A.R.E. Clinic, it was our routine, when

a pregnant woman started to have any kind of difficulty to apply a castor oil pack to her abdomen. If there was any sign of threatened spontaneous abortion, we would have the mother go to bed, elevate the foot of the bed, and put a pack on—without the heating pad—and often she would then carry the pregnancy on to term.

When a pregnant woman who had a history of miscarriages would come to the clinic, the castor oil pack would be the primary and immediate therapy. There are teenagers and young adults walking around throughout the Phoenix area who may not have made it to birthing had it not been for the use of the castor oil packs. And mothers who used the packs noted also that there were few stretch marks, if indeed any appeared.

Because of my extensive writing about my work with the Cayce material and castor oil over the past twenty years, many users of the Cayce suggestions write me about their experiences. One forty-year-old man volunteered his story about intermittent pain that he had suffered since he was eighteen. It was irritating, but not disabling. After reading about the use of castor oil in other conditions, he decided to try it. The pain was in the center of each wrist. He applied a pack to each wrist all night long for three consecutive nights. When he wrote to me—more than three months after his treatment, he said he had had the pain "since I was eighteen years old, and I'm now forty—and the pain has not returned since I used the packs." He added that he had experienced some pain in his upper arm. Using the packs also cleared up that pain with no recurrence.

I'm sure there were reasons for the occurrence of the pain in this man's case and he would need to become aware of what really lay behind his pain episode. It was obvious, however, that this man had a castor oil consciousness.

We have used castor oil on the body in a variety of locations, and the doctors who have been on the staff of the

Clinic have become strong advocates for its use, as have many of our patients and correspondents.

Before he retired, Dr. Ray Bjork sent me this report: "I have been seeing a man who complains of tinnitus, a ringing in the ears. Acupuncture has helped only mildly so far. But he had a keratotic (wart-like) lesion on his forearm and wanted to know if he should see a skin specialist as he wondered if it might be cancerous. I told him I felt it was benign but gave him a dermatologist's address. Before he left the office, I applied a Band-Aid® with drops of castor oil on it and told him to apply one drop twice a day.

"It ended up that he did not go to the specialist, and the lesion sloughed off in just a couple of weeks."

Chapter Six
Therapists Are Born, Not Made

WHEN INDIVIDUALS WITH NO MEDICAL TRAINING FIND OUT about very simple therapies that are harmless but very interesting and have a history of being helpful, some become fascinated. They want to know "What happens if . . . ?" These are therapists who are born that way. I suspect that they have had past lives helping other humans through physical or mental difficulties.

When I was in Virginia Beach several years ago, an A.R.E. member told me about a friend of hers who must have been one of these "born-again" therapists. She worked at a supermarket checkout counter, but loved the use of castor oil and most of the Cayce remedies. She would tell her customers about these things as they checked out. Most of the time her customers do nothing about her suggestions, but on those occasions when they do, they get results.

One woman came through her checkout counter who had plastic wrapped around one leg and was obviously uncomfortable. Emma, the checkout clerk, said, "What in the world happened to your leg?" The answer, "Varicose veins!" The skin had broken down and would not heal no matter what she did. She had even spent three months in bed with no results. Emma told her about soaking a cloth in castor oil and wrapping it around her leg underneath the plastic. She didn't tell her anything else.

Emma saw the lady's husband about a month later and asked how his wife was doing. His answer, "You know, after two or three weeks, the leg healed up completely, and she's had no trouble with it since."

Another one of those investigative therapists was a patient of mine, who told me his story after the fact. He severely sprained his ankle. He wrote this account and sent it to me: "I used castor oil Saturday and Sunday nights and I am amazed at what it does. When I talked with you, I had just had the pack on for about half an hour and had gone to bed to keep my foot up. The pain was pretty hard to take, but after we were through on the telephone, I went back to bed and within a half hour the pain left almost suddenly, and I never had a recurrence.

"I slept like a log, put my foot in any position I wished, and could walk on it the next morning by using chairs along the way. Two nights before I couldn't even step on it. I had to hang on to things and shuffle my good foot back and forth on the rug until I got to the phone . . . Now my ankle is fine, discolored a bit but no swelling, and I bind it up and go on my way."

In the early days of my association with the Cayce material, I was on call for the emergency room at one of the local hospitals. A woman who had sprained her ankle at work had been taken to the emergency room. X-rays showed no fracture. I checked her ankle; it was swollen and tender to pressure and she had difficulty bearing weight on that foot. I instructed her to make up a castor oil pack and wear it constantly for the next two days, using an elastic bandage to hold it in place and to provide some pressure to keep the swelling down.

Two days later she appeared at our office, walking normally, with the pack in place. When I checked her ankle, she told me that my instructions were so strange that when she got out of the hospital, she thought, "What am I doing? That's the craziest thing I ever heard of!" But, she said, since she didn't have anything else to do and her ankle was hurting, she followed the instructions.

She used an elastic bandage for the next few days, but she walked without a limp and there was no pain. Even I was surprised at that kind of dramatic response. It represents more evidence for me on the amazing value of a common substance used to bring new awareness to the forces within the human body.

Many other experiences come from among our patient population and from those who correspond with me, but this one tells the story in a different way:

This was another instance in which a woman suffered a nasty sprain to her ankle. She knew about using castor oil packs and she put one together at once, applying the pack warm, covering the ankle and the foot, and using a plastic baggie to cover both.

The ankle hurt "like blazes," she said, for about two hours, but then the pain disappeared completely. She used crutches the first day, but discarded them after that, keeping the pack on day and night for three days, warming it occasionally. Her ankle was a bit tender for a few days, but she was off it for just the first day.

Her husband had sprained his ankle years ago and was disabled and on crutches for three weeks. More recently a friend of hers was six weeks on crutches after her ankle was sprained. When they talked together (six weeks after the injury), the friend's ankle was still swollen and painful. She took the suggestion, however, about using the packs and reported that she was delighted with the results.

INJURIES AND ABRASIONS

Because of the as-yet-unexplained healing qualities in castor oil, we have used it extensively with our patients, the personnel at the Clinic, and in our own lives. We have found that any puncture wound clears up almost immediately simply by applying castor oil over the area gently several times a day. The date palm trees in our back yard rarely got a trimming without my getting one or two puncture wounds from the needle-like ends of the fronds. I found out years ago that these wounds would become irritated and infected, if left unattended. I used to apply antibiotic cream on them, but that wasn't helpful. When I discovered the efficacy of castor oil, I never had an infected puncture wound again. I would rub castor oil into the area after washing it, repeat it again several hours later, and then again at bedtime. If it was still reminding me that it was not feeling good in the morning, I would apply the oil once again. Usually, this would take care of the problem.

Our six children have had castor oil applied to various parts of their anatomy so often over the years that they have reminded us that they will put on our tombstones when we die, "Here they lie in spite of castor oil!"

The experience paid off in our caring for our patients and friends, and—as I mentioned earlier—it led to my writing a monograph about the use of castor oil packs in the practice of medicine. It developed into a book and acquired its name because someone in the Middle Ages called the castor bean plant the *Palma Christi*, the palm of Christ.[8]

A patient of ours, Sherri, was traveling about forty-five miles per hour on her motorbike when she lost control and crashed. Sherri had skin abrasions on her elbows, abdomen, and left breast, and the palms of both hands were scraped raw down to the dermal layer. Her therapy was castor oil, used liberally on all the affected areas. Her response was excellent. The wounds healed completely without scars.

Injuries at birth sometimes come in the form of bleeding under the skin of the scalp, which is called a hematoma (a tumor filled with blood). This is what happened when Patti's third son was born. The tumor was relatively small right after birth, but continued to grow in size until the baby was two months old. At that point, it was the size of a baseball, and it was then that the mother started using a castor oil pack on his head, keeping it in place with the ingenuity born of motherhood.

It rapidly decreased in size and, within the next ten days, the hematoma was no longer present.

We have treated fingernails that had been "smashed," using a little pack kept in place with a Band-Aid®. If treated early enough, the blackened nail gradually gains back its normal color and the blood is reabsorbed.

ELIMINATIONS USING CASTOR OIL

I gradually became aware of another healing concept after seeing the efficiency of castor oil in resolving bleeding in the tissues and exciting the rebuilding of tissues after serious injury to the skin. The concept: that elimination internally and regeneration of the tissue are primary effects when castor oil is applied to the body. If this principle is exercised in therapy, much can be accomplished in the body's healing process.

Too little attention is given to the importance of eliminations in the medical world today. It is physiologically true that there are four channels of elimination in the body: the skin, the lungs, the kidneys, and the liver/intestinal tract. When one channel is obstructed, damaged, or ill and unable to do its job, the other three suffer. And the body is much the worse for wear.

When an eliminatory organ or system can be returned to a more normal state, the body benefits. Thus, any method designed to improve and coordinate the eliminations of the body is bound to be helpful to its recovery.

It must be kept in mind that the lymphatics and capillaries are important in transferring substances that need to be removed from where they might be found in the body.

Proper eliminations provide a greater degree of cleanliness to the cells within the body. Being clean internally, the cells function more efficiently and lend themselves to the healing or maintenance of health in the body as a whole. It's probably wise to remember that in the Bible we are told that cleanliness is next to godliness.

TUMOR IN THE NECK

Catherine, a young eighty-two, had been thriving under the various therapies suggested in the Edgar Cayce readings. She paid me a visit at the Clinic some time ago because she had developed a lump in the right side of her neck near the angle of her mandible (jaw bone) very close to the attachment of the earlobe.

There was no evidence of any difficulty that would cause a lymph node in that area to be enlarged, so x-rays and laboratory tests were ordered. Still, no basic cause was uncovered.

When she discovered the lump prior to the office call, Catherine began applying castor oil packs to that area. When we first saw the lump, it was the size of a hazelnut and quite firm. In two weeks' time, the size was down to that of a small pea, and one month later the lump was gone.

Looking back at the event, I suspect it was a lymph node. Had it not rapidly decreased in size, I would have advised a biopsy, a procedure she may have rejected. But no cause was demonstrated and the patient exited from the event in excellent health. In this instance, we did not know what was going on, but we opted to take steps to return the body back to normal. And the castor oil did it.

"HORNY" TOE NAIL

This is a rather common problem in the practice of family medicine, but it is very difficult to correct. Removal does not often provide a cure. It is felt that a fungus may be the etiology, the cause. It is most common in the elderly. In 1977 a woman presented her big toe as a problem for us to solve. It was the site of a "horny" toe nail, large, angled, and very difficult to trim or keep under control.

She was instructed to use foot soaks of Epsom salt for fifteen minutes every night at bedtime. Then she was to wrap the toe in a small castor oil pack, which was to be kept on all night long. This procedure was to be continued for two months. She was seen just six months later. Upon examination, we found her nail to be completely normal.

What happened? Increased circulation? Better lymphatic flow? Fungicidal activity? Faith? Patience and persistence? How her toe nail responded remains—like many other physiological responses—an enigma. But, with patience, persistence, consistency, and castor oil she fixed it!

SKIN CANCER/KERATOSIS

In the early stages, it is probably impossible to tell whether an actinic keratosis is going to develop into what is called a keratotic horn or a squamous cell carcinoma, which is malignant. Commonly, these excessive growths of epidermal cells, keratinocytes, are usually called keratoses. Often, even without a biopsy to prove the point, they are called early or advanced skin cancers. Non-physicians often make the diagnoses themselves.

A woman from Boulder, Colorado, wrote me about her experience: "I had a skin cancer on my nose, near my right eye, which has disappeared after three days of applying castor oil first, then sprinkling baking soda over the spot! I had had the cancer for two years, trying every natural method I had read or heard about. I had previously tried castor oil and a small amount of baking soda in a mixture with no success."

One of my favorite patients is ninety-three years old (his wife is ninety-five). Both have a tremendous sense of humor. George had a large growth on his right earlobe—a keratosis—which was disfiguring, although not malignant. He had been treated by several other doctors before I saw him, but the keratosis persisted. I instructed him to rub castor oil thoroughly on the earlobe twice daily, and clean it off with a soft cloth. After he returned a year and a half later, the ear was completely normal—no keratosis. He was still using the castor oil, he reported, because it made his ear feel so soft.

An out-of-town friend wrote us about her experience with a similar difficulty. "For about ten years I had a large keratosis (diagnosed by a dermatologist) on each side of my face just in front of the ears. They were removed by the doctor—the one on the right was treated surgically three times—yet both enlarged again each time after treatment. So I just lived with them until finally I realized they were both spreading.

"I began saturating them with castor oil on cotton, covered with a Band-Aid®. I did this every night and noticed that they were changing in color and size. The center parts began erupting, scabbing over, then peeling off—until finally, after about a five-month period, they were both completely gone! The skin is now smooth with no scars that can be seen."

We have routinely advised our patients to use castor oil on the skin for keratoses, for acne, stretch marks in pregnancy, and general care of the skin. One of our patients rubbed castor oil on her abdomen to prevent stretch marks, and then, noticing that she was developing acne, added treatment to those lesions to her skin-care routine. The acne cleared up and her face was so smooth that she told us that people took her for being twenty-three or twenty-four instead of thirty-five—her real age.

INFECTION AFTER INJURY

Jeff Asher, the son of a longtime friend, lived with us during a good portion of his university studies. We became fast friends and have shared many experiences. His mother Jenny told me a story many years ago and then followed it up with a letter because she was so deeply involved with the Cayce work. Her experience is the kind of thing that happens to people as they come to sudden—or gradual—awareness about something they know but have not yet made real in this world by putting it into action.

"When my daughter, Jody, was twelve, the children were playing on the road. Their ball went down a sewer covered by a manhole cover. The children pried up the heavy, filthy cover but it fell down again on Jody's bare toes. Her big toe and the next two were crushed.

"We rushed her to UCLA emergency center. An orthopedic surgeon was called in. He cleaned it up as best he could and instructed me to soak it four times a day in Epsom salt solutions and to use a Q-tip® each time to clean around the nailbeds. She was put on antibiotics.

"Four months and three orthopedic surgeons later—one wanted to do a debriding (removing foreign matter and devitalized tissue) in the hospital, which would also shorten her toe—she was on crutches. Her toes would swell with pus every few days. She was still on antibiotics.

"I had your book on the Palma Christi. There is a case of a

man who dropped a drum of tar on his foot. Cayce recommended castor oil. The man, I believe, was back in shoes and at work in a matter of weeks. But it takes a whole different brand of courage to defy doctor's orders when it concerns your own child and not you yourself. I didn't have the courage, at first. Finally, one Sunday afternoon, I was soaking her foot as usual and could see it was again swelling with pus. This was after four months of the trouble. It was a painful, awful mess. We had an appointment with the doctor on the next Wednesday. I decided to risk the castor oil and simply poured it on from the bottle. The toes could not have tolerated flannel or a pack. Epsom salt soaks and the Q-tip® cleaning were stopped. Just the castor oil.

"On Wednesday, we went to the orthopedic surgeon's office, your Palma Christi book in hand. I told Jody not to say anything to the doctor. We would wait to hear what he would say. Well, he looked at the toes and said, 'We sure cleaned it up this time!'

"I then told him what we had done and handed him the Palma Christi book and he read that case. He handed it back to me, shook his head, and said, 'I don't care if it's mud. It worked!'

"Well, Jody's toes healed quickly after that. She never grew the nail on the large toe and the toe is a bit deformed. I am sorry I waited four months to try the castor oil. I'll bet her nail would have grown in, too."

There are castor oil proponents throughout the United States, and I hear from many of them. One is an owner of a clock shop, but I suspect he sells more castor oil than clocks. He had such good results himself by soaking a pair of socks in castor oil and wearing them with an old pair of shoes (his problem was aching feet) that he told a friend about his methods. His friend worked in a factory and was on his feet on the hard concrete all day long—and his feet ached, too. He didn't say anything to his friends at that point, but his results in developing happy feet were so resounding that he told the clock-shop man that he spread the word around and "You can hear the sloshing of castor oil feet nearly everywhere in the factory."

We learn about simple things in many ways, and the seed is planted for growth in awareness.

HYPERACTIVITY

Much has been written about this affliction which also has the name or is associated with what is called dyslexia, an impairment of the ability to read. One lesson I've learned over the years is to look at the deeper causation of problems rather than the end product of a process.

The development of physiological abnormalities is the process. On the causative side of this process are those factors that create the abnormalities. On the resultant side of the same process is the manifestation, which is termed a disease or syndrome. Everything in the human body is changing for the better or for the worse as life continues, and we are always creating at the level of the mind and the emotions. This creative activity impacts the physiology for better or for worse.

In this instance, hyperactivity was the end product. The deeper problem must lie somewhere in the relationship among the activity of the mind, the emotional nature, and the neurological impulses which either bring information into our consciousness or cause the body to act. This places the cause, then, directly inside the nervous system.

It's truly interesting to let the creative part of yourself loose and consider that the same application which helps a man stop snoring and become a cooperative instead of an antagonistic individual might also have a beneficial effect on hyperactivity. Both conditions lie in the realm of the autonomic nervous system.

This kind of speculation does not currently reside in the scientific field, but it might indeed have a reality if we acknowledge that most of the nature of humanity cannot be quantified, but has its ultimate meaning in a spiritual realm about which we know very little.

I recall one woman, in her late fifties, who reported to me that the castor oil pack which she had put on for the very first time was the best tranquilizer she had ever used. Others have told me that it helps them sleep, it relaxes them, and it soothes them. One might say it helps to normalize the body when applied over the abdomen, where the solar plexus is to be found—the largest accumulations of autonomic nerve cells in the lower part of the body.

It was in 1960 that we had our first real encounter with severe hyperactivity. Tommy's mother told about his lifelong problem while she picked up torn magazines that Tommy had worked over, pushed drawers back in place in the examining room, pulled Tommy from the tops of furniture time and again—trying to restore order where he was creating chaos. He was everywhere and could not be quieted down.

He was in our office for a mild belly ache. The hyperactivity was a daily occurrence to which his mother had adapted. Mother was instructed to use a castor oil pack for the abdominal problem and to bring Tommy back if he was not doing well.

The next visit, three weeks later, was a revelation. Tommy was quiet, sat on a chair reading a book, turning the pages without tearing them out, answering questions like the average child, and showing no signs of hyperactivity.

What was happening? Every evening, his mother placed the castor oil pack on Tommy's abdomen while he was watching television. She didn't like having him watch television but she knew he would stay quiet. In a few days, he started reminding his mother to put the pack on because it felt so good. Her life was changed. Tommy was no longer a threat to the sanity of his parents nor to the furniture, wallpaper, or glassware. He was a normal five-year-old boy getting ready to go to school.

Ever since that experience, we have been treating hyperactivity with a good diet and castor oil packs, not with medication. Tommy grew up, got married, and now brings his kids in for a checkup occasionally. There is no hyperactivity now in that family.

THE LIVER AND GALL BLADDER

Part of my awareness of the healing qualities of substances offered us by Mother Nature came about as I watched one kind of disturbance of the body after another respond to the application of a castor oil pack. We first used the packs on hepatitis because of the frequency with which Cayce, in his readings, suggested that they would be beneficial. Gall bladder conditions received much the same sort of attention in the readings.

Consistently, through the thirty years I have worked with the Cayce information, the use of castor oil packs for liver and gall bladder conditions has remained our standard. Rarely, if ever, have they failed to perform advantageously.

A nursing student, recognizing the onset of hepatitis, took a week off, loaded up with water and more water, and wore a castor oil pack continuously. She also had people pray for her. The following Monday she returned to school with no sign of the yellowish tint to her skin or conjunctivae of the eyes. The diagnosis had been confirmed early in the course of her illness, so there was no question about its validity. She would not have been able to continue in her training if she had missed more school than she did.

In 1978, we began a residential seventeen-day Temple Beautiful Program, fashioned to an extent after the ancient

Temple Beautiful described in the Edgar Cayce readings. Later on, it became an eleven-day event, providing patients with a healing experience, linking together the body, mind, and spirit portions of the human being.

Joel Buchanan, a patient of ours who earlier had been through one of these programs, called me from Texas for some advice. He wanted to keep his liver in good shape. Early in 1987, he developed type B hepatitis, which he treated at home with castor oil packs. He was seeing his internist but didn't tell him what he was doing because he felt the packs would be discredited by the doctor.

He had, however, a rapid recovery and his internist kept saying that his return to health was "miraculous," considering his sixty-six years and the severity of the case. I told him that the same therapy that helped his liver back to health would help it maintain its health. So he continued using the packs periodically.

A correspondent, Richard Garcia, called me more than two years ago about the gallstones that had been discovered in his gall bladder. He had been doing a three-day apple diet and took olive oil by mouth on the third day. This diet he had continued intermittently for many years. But he was still having episodes of pain and discomfort. He knew about castor oil packs but had not used them, and he was discouraged. I told him that surgery was always an alternative.

His letter came quite recently letting me know that he had gone ahead and scheduled himself to see the surgeon: "But when I met with the surgeon he told me that there was a nerve that ran close by the gall bladder that they couldn't avoid cutting. That really turned me off, so I got really serious and started a three-month, five-days-on, three-days-off series of castor oil packs. On the fifth evening after each series, I drank a half-cup of olive oil. The treatment did wonders for me and I had had no recurrences." (Garcia decided on a half-cup of olive oil on his on. Cayce, as far as I know, never recommended that much oil in one dose. More commonly, it was a tablespoonful.)

Garcia did not tell me whether he had passed the stones or if he had taken another x-ray of his gall bladder, but his pain and discomfort no longer gave him trouble, and he has continued occasionally to use a three-day series of packs to help "balance" his body.

ESOPHAGEAL SPASM

It is sometimes astonishing even to me—since I have utilized castor oil packs in a variety of conditions over the last thirty years in my practice—to hear how some of my correspondents have used this kind of aid for the body. Not long ago I received a letter from a man I've known for a long time. He's a Texan, so I don't get to see him often. He wanted to touch base with me and report something that happened to him back in 1979.

He reports: "I was having problems with my esophagus and was having it dilated about every six weeks to two months. You suggested the castor oil packs, so I came home from the conference and started using them pretty religiously for the rest of that year and into the next. I have not had to return for a dilation since and don't expect to ever again. I want to thank you!"

Where did he use them? Over the abdomen and sometimes directly over the chest where the spasm was located. The healing process always amazes me, and I am convinced over and over again that healing is just about like making the right turn in a road that leads to the destination desired.

EAR PROBLEMS / HEARING LOSS

More than a year ago, I received a letter from Sharon Roznik telling me about the plight of her two-year-old boy, who "has had fluid trapped in his ear tubes for six months." They had an appointment with an ear doctor who was planning on placing drainage tubes in his ears. She wanted to know what Edgar Cayce would have suggested, because she believed that there must be a better way to get fluid out of Jesse's ears.

By the time she received my answer, she had taken action and had already seen the doctor. Her story in response to my letter is provocative:

"Guess what! I just played it by 'ear,' giving him 250 mg. of vitamin C; castor oil drops in ears a.m. and p.m.; high-alkaline, low-acid diet; a couple drops of Glyco-Thymoline (see Appendix) orally every few days; castor oil soaked on the front of his diaper at bedtime; upper back massages; laying on of hands (mine) with white healing light in mind. He wouldn't tolerate Glyco-Thymoline packs to the neck! I started this ten days before he was to see the ear specialist. By the way, Jesse was going in because he's had fluid in his ears for six months straight, without any signs of clearing up, after taking various antibiotics and decongestants, and being checked regularly by a doctor every three weeks.

"When the ear doctor looked in Jesse's ears, my husband said there was a look of shock on his face. His right ear was completely clear and his left still had some fluid remaining in it. I was so relieved and grateful.

"The doctor asked if he'd been on any medication this past month and I said 'no.' I don't know why I said that. Next time I go in (in five weeks to check the other ear) I'll tell him.

"I realize that tubes in the ears aren't really a serious health threat, but I just felt deep inside my heart that a little boy shouldn't have to have tubes put in his ears. There should be a natural way to get fluid out of those ears.

"Thank you for the book, *The Edgar Cayce Remedies*,[9] where I found the answer to this health problem. This is the first time I ever tried an extensive remedy like this. Thanks for answering my letter, and thank God for simple truths!"

I've always thought that simple truths are the best. After all, if we are destined to be one with Creative Forces and if there's a oneness among all of humankind, then there may be little that can be more basic than the simple truths.

Hearing loss can come from a variety of causes, but it is always a barrier to full participation in life as it is lived on this planet. When an eight-year-old boy is afflicted, we may not think that it is as detrimental to him as to an adult, because he can adjust better. However, we seldom listen carefully to such a person to see what *he* thinks of the problem. Loss of hearing, partial or complete, is a real problem to anyone.

Jonathan had such a problem, but his solution—thanks to his mother and some ideas from the Cayce material—was a happy one. This is from his mother's letter:

"My son Jonathan, age eight, has had tubes put in his ears twice. The last time was about two years ago and in one ear he has not heard well for about a year and a half. (I knew this because he couldn't hear the buzz tone on the telephone.) I followed the Cayce instructions of massage, head and neck exercise, and the lamb tallow mixture for four evenings. Then, the next evening I put a drop of castor oil in his ear. The following morning, I looked in his ear and the tube had fallen out! One side of the tube looked fine, but the other side was crusted over with dried blood! . . . needless to say, I am thrilled to report that he now hears normally in both ears! God answered my prayers."

In our work with the Cayce readings and the concepts of healing found there, we ventured outward to use castor oil in a number of ways that would either activate the immune system or quiet down the autonomic nervous system. We found that castor oil drops in the ears would often take care of minor problems there and sometimes influence major difficulties toward healing.

A California woman wrote to me about her experience with a problem of minimal hearing loss: "About three months ago I noticed my hearing diminishing in my left ear. I had several colds, plus my travels take me up and down a mountain to get to work.

"A month and a half ago I went to an ear, nose, and throat specialist who gave me some strong decongestant tablets and a spray. Those dried up my cold and sinuses and somewhat relieved the problem, but not completely. I went back and he punctured my eardrum and blew medication into it to loosen and help drain the tube. It helped for two days, but then my hearing worsened again. I decided to use castor oil packs directly on the ear, with heat, at night when going to bed—I used them for one hour.

"After the first treatment, I was much improved and after the second night there was very little hearing loss." No long-term report on this, but when one experiences the kind of benefits she felt in her own body, it excites her and opens her mind to the concept that the body indeed can be helped toward a better level of homeostasis, a condition we call health.

SNORING

We are all familiar with it and many of us do it. It is defined as rough, noisy breathing during sleep, due to vibration of the uvula and soft palate. Some husbands and perhaps more wives suffer insomnia when their spouses snore. But there is a story that I remember reading about a woman who had just been married back in the Depression era. The newlyweds took residence in the second-floor apartment of a rickety wood building. As her husband fell asleep, she began to hear the sound of rats or mice in the walls of their apartment, and she was terrified. Then her husband began to snore, and the rodents ceased their movement. As long as he was snoring, the rats were quiet.

She has associated snoring ever since with peace and tranquillity, and, I suppose to her, it was like the sound of the waves would be to others who live by the ocean.

Snoring was the subject of several questions given the sleeping Cayce. They provide another perspective on this condition:

(Q) Is there any way of sleeping on the back without snoring?
(A) Not that has been invented yet! (1861-18)

(Q) May anything be done to correct or prevent sleeping with mouth open?
(A) Close it!
(Q) When asleep, how may this be done?
(A) Make the suggestions to self as going to sleep. Get the system balanced. And this will be done. (288-41)

In the early 1930s, Edgar Cayce and a group of devoted individuals worked together to write a book called *A Search for God.*[10] It has become the guiding light for thousands of people since that time as they join together in study groups once a week.

From a study group member comes a story of a unique application of castor oil packs. It seems that this young woman's mother and dad were at the point of sleeping in separate rooms because of his snoring so that the wife could get some sleep. The daughter wrote me: "My parents are both sleeping better now, thanks to the castor oil pack. My mother has insisted that dad wear a pack every night for the last two weeks.

"Now, instead of her being kept awake by loud guttural, choking snores and frequent angry outcries originating from nightly dreams of fighting, the snoring has ceased totally and she is occasionally awakened by the most soft, whimsical giggling coming from the original offender—my dad! Mom also reports an enhanced sense of humor, a very affectionate husband, and a spirit of cooperation that just won't quit."

Psychotherapy? I would think not, unless we were to define that word a bit differently. In the field of endocrinology, the adrenal gland is called the "fight/flight" gland and is symbolized in the texts by a man, crouched with his fists ready, eyes wide, alert, and prepared for combat or for running—if that seems to be the best course to take.

This kind of response by the adrenal gland excited my wonderment once more. Why should a pack placed on the abdomen alter the emotional nature (and dream patterns) of an adult person? Did these packs actually create within the consciousness of the adrenal gland and the accompanying sympathetic nervous system a more peaceable vibration? Jesus said, "Peace is my parting gift to you, my own peace, such as the world cannot give. Set your troubled hearts at rest, and banish your fears."[11] And the castor bean plant was called the *Palma Christi* (the palm of Christ) several hundred years ago.

THE PALMA CHRISTI

Our youngest son, David—who is now a physician—lived a great deal of his life in close companionship with his guardian angels. He must have had more than one angel. When visiting an old college classmate of mine in Santa Rosa, California, we were enjoying our conversation in the living room after dinner, while the two boys (David and Garrick) were climbing up and down the outside of the stairs in the split-level home. They would climb up to the landing, then drop to the stairs below that led down to the family room.

It was getting late, and we thought it was time for the kids to go to bed. I announced this to David, and he said, "One more time, Dad!" So up he climbed, one more time, but this time he was holding onto the landing above and was swinging back and forth before dropping. He swung too far, and his fingers slipped off the landing floor. With a thud, he landed on his back on the stairs below—and he let out a scream. I was there in no time, picked him up, and carried him over to the living room floor where he could be checked for possible serious injury.

His back was hurting badly and was very tender to the touch, but there was no evidence of neurological injury. X-rays could wait till morning, and he slept on the floor alongside the bed the rest of the night.

With a castor oil pack on his back, David slept very fitfully until about four in the morning, when he finally fell sound asleep. In the morning, he was still asleep. Eventually I checked him for problems. He said he had no pain, so I palpated the injured area. It was not tender. I had him sit up, then stand up, bend this way and that, and it was as if nothing had happened to him. It was then that he told us that he had a dream. "I was lying there with my back hurting for a long time, and then Jesus came and put His hand on my back and the pain stopped."

What kind of healing vibration is there in castor oil that would inspire someone to call the plant the palm of the Christ, the Palma Christi? This happened back in the Middle Ages.[12] And how could this relate to the dream—the sleeping consciousness—of an eight-year-old boy so that he would recognize Jesus putting His palm on his back and healing him?

From snoring to giggling; from discord to cooperation; from pain to healing—let's keep on unfolding the mystery of this wonderful creation—the human being—whom God created in some inexplicable manner. Let's keep on smelling the dandelions.

Chapter Seven
Why Castor Oil?

WE STILL HAVE NO EXPLANATION WHY CAS-
TOR OIL placed in the ear canal will be so helpful to a child
with a hearing problem, or why a pack using this oil will
help restore normalcy to a hyperactive child, or speed up
the healing of hepatitis, or help to get rid of gallstones, or
even help heal abrasions and infections. Perhaps it is to be
found in the nature of the human body and the secret healing capabilities of the substances God gave us here on the
earth for our use and benefit.

In his sleeping state, Cayce saw illness in the human being as the end point of malfunctioning physiology. Thus, in
an attempt to correct the ailing body, the suggestions were
aimed at the functioning parts—the physiology—not at the
end point of a process. This is a very important distinction,
for it indicates the difference between the manner in which
Cayce looked at this individual created in the image of God
and the manner in which I was taught to search for a diag-

nosis and, in a sense, forget about the human being whose physiology created the problem in the first place.

Cayce described at least thirty different physiological functions that were changed for the better through the use of castor oil applied topically, mostly by the use of the packs.[13] Here's a partial list, in Cayce's unique language and based on his understanding of the internal workings of the body:

> Increases eliminations
> Stimulates the liver
> Dissolves and removes adhesions
> Dissolves and removes lesions
> Relieves pain
> Releases colon impaction
> Reduces nervous system
> Stimulates the gall bladder
> Incoordinations reducing toxemia
> Reduces flatulence
> Increases lymphatic circulation
> Improves intestinal assimilation
> Balances eliminations
> Reduces inflammation
> Increases relaxation
> Dissolves lacteal duct adhesions
> Reduces nausea
> Dissolves gallstones
> Stimulates lacteal duct circulation
> Reduces swelling
> Stimulates the caecum
> Coordinates liver-kidney function
> Stimulates organs and glands

Based on the above list, it is understandable that castor oil packs were advocated in the readings as therapy for people who had been diagnosed with a variety of bodily conditions:

aphonia	appendicitis	arthritis
cancer	cholecystitis	cholecystalgia
colitis	constipation	epilepsy
gallstones	gastritis	migraine
hepatitis	hernia	Hodgkin's disease
hookworm	intestinal impaction	sluggish liver
stenosis of the duodenum	stricture of duodenum	strangulation of kidneys
neuritis	cirrhosis of liver	multiple sclerosis
lymphitis	cerebral palsy	pelvic cellulitis
uremia	sterility	ringworm
Parkinson's disease		

This list does not include a multitude of cases indexed in the A.R.E. Library at Virginia Beach as: "lesions, incoordinations, intestines, toxemia, eliminations, and adhesions."[14]

This oil that heals, of course, is that which is extracted from the seed of the *Ricinus communis*, known also—as mentioned before—as the Palma Christi or more commonly as the castor oil plant. This is what Edgar Cayce recommended for use so very, very frequently in the form of a pack.

It is probable that Cleopatra used castor oil as a base for her make-up or to make even more lovely her eyes, just as this particular oil is found commonly in lipstick and make-up today, presumably because of its stable and soothing characteristics. In the Ebers Papyrus (ca. 1550 B.C.), castor oil was described as being used as eyedrops to protect the eyes from irritation.[15] So we see perhaps the beginning of the recorded use of this unusual oil as therapy in ancient Egypt, a land shrouded in many mysteries.

Over the centuries, the value of castor oil continued to be recognized, sometimes in new ways, but the real nature of its action as described in the Cayce readings remained an enigma. An exhaustive search of medical literature going back forty-nine years produced few but fascinating references.

Douglas W. Montgomery, M.D., wrote in 1918 of the oil which he described as coming from a beautiful plant with large palmate leaves, often called Palma Christi, the palm of the Christ.[16] Somewhat facetiously, I suspect, he said, "If as a child I had known this sonorous name, it might have mitigated the misery I often suffered in having to take the oil. A very determined and energetic Scotch auntie regarded 'a crumb o' oil,' as she used to call it, as a universal remedy of exceeding potency in both moral and physical contingencies; and indeed, there is no doubt of its efficiency as a cleaner."

Montgomery did report in the same paper an observation which is of interest and importance today to physicians and which correlates with some of the commentaries made in the Cayce readings about the use of castor oil. He observed that in diseases of the skin, the use of castor oil is of importance inasmuch as a clean alimentary canal is conducive to a clean cutaneous surface. "It would appear that the medicine acts particularly on the ascending colon, and this is interesting, as it is undoubtedly a fact that many of the more active skin reactions are caused by poisons generated in caput coli, a favorable location for the anaerobic proteolytic bacteria." He further pointed out that in the work W. B. Cannon reported on,[17] in which castor oil was given to an animal with its food, there was a serial sectioning of the food in the ascending colon followed each time by antiperistalsis which swept the food back—a type of action well fitted to clear out the haustra of the colon, "those pockets which in colonic sluggishness must tend to become especially dirty."

Important findings are often disregarded even in our most astute textbooks. Here is evidence of ascending colon activity as a direct result of the castor oil taken internally. Goodman and Gilman[18] tell how the oil is hydrolyzed by the fat-splitting enzymes in the small intestine into glycerol and ricinoleic acid. It is the latter substance which is active in producing catharsis (a purging), through its marked irritant activity in stimulating the motor activity (parasympathetic) of the intestines to promote rapid propulsion of the contents of the small intestine. Then the text states that "the colon is stimulated little, for in passage through the small intestine the ricinoleic acid is absorbed just as are other fatty acids."

The activity which Cannon reported on is most likely a reflex-type phenomenon called irradiation (the dispersion of a nervous impulse beyond the normal path of conduction). In such an event, it would be understandable how the castor oil would act as a stimulant to the entire small intestine and the ascending half of the transverse colon through the spread of impulses resulting from the irritant activity.

In the autonomic nervous system, irradiation is a much more pronounced phenomenon than in the central nervous system.[19] Indeed, as regards the sympathetic system, the effect of an afferent impulse (toward an organ or part) is to set the whole sympathetic system into activity, and its structure is well suited for such widespread responses. Hence, for example, if the central end of the splanchnic (visceral) nerve is stimulated, the effects reach even to the pupil, which dilates. In the parasympathetic system there is less irradiation than in the sympathetic, but it still is well marked.

Thus the effect of the castor oil is seen in the colon before it proceeds even a small distance through the small bowel, through the effect of irradiation. It illustrates the fact that there are many functions happening in this wonderful human body of ours that are more delicate and more mysterious than we, at our present stage of knowledge, truly understand.

Among the historical notes is a study[20] reported in the *Southern Medical Journal* by a dermatologist covering his study of ten cases of skin eruption treated with castor oil or sodium ricinoleate internally. Apparently, Schoch had read Cannon's report and he put that information together with a concept he shared with other dermatologists of the thirties that toxins loculated in the caput or head of the ascending colon were absorbed and created dermatological problems. Cannon's observations then led him to test the theory that cleansing of that part of the colon would lead to clearing of the skin.

When he tested it in the ten cases he reported, the results were sometimes quite remarkable. One instance was a thirty-year-old graduate nurse who had severe bath pruritis (itching) of four years' duration. She had failed to improve under generalized ultraviolet light, I.V. calcium gluconate and sodium iodide, elimination diets, autohemotherapy, and local therapy. She had not risked a tub or shower bath in seven months.

Dr. Schoch placed her on kaolin and sodium ricinoleate by mouth, half an ounce three times daily. Four days later she reported that she was well, had bought some soap, and was taking four baths a day. After a short recurrence six months later which responded to the same therapy, there had been no recurrence in two and a half years.

Another case he presented was that of a seventy-two-year-old man with a non-exudative urticarial dermatitis involving the back, arms, and legs. It had lasted for two weeks. The man was given a single dose of castor oil by mouth without any other therapy. The pruritis subsided in twenty-four hours, and the rash cleared up in one week.

Pharmacologically, castor oil is known to be composed mostly of ricinoleic acid, an unsaturated hydroxy fatty acid with the formula $CH_3(CH_2)_5CHOHCH_2CH: CH(CH_2)_7COOH$. It's known in Goodman and Gilman[21] as a bland emollient and is employed locally on the skin for its soothing properties. Castor oil is also incorporated with alcohol and extensively used as a hair tonic, in the proportions of one part of oil to ten of alcohol.

Ormsby and Montgomery[22] describe castor oil as one of the "nutritive and soothing oils" which may be used by direct application or through saturated compresses to the skin. These are frequently used for the removal of crusts and scales. Interestingly, the other "nutritive and soothing oils" which the authors list are cod-liver, olive, almond, linseed, and neat's foot, while the "stimulating" oils are those of tar, cade, white birch, cashew-nut, and juniper.

Chemically, castor oil is a triglyceride (ester) of fatty acids. It is unique in that approximately ninety percent of this fatty acid content is ricinoleic acid, and eighteen-carbon acid having a double bond in the nine-to-ten position and a hydroxyl group on the twelfth carbon. *This relationship of hydroxyl group and unsaturation exists only in castor oil.*[23] The typical composition of castor oil fatty acids is shown below. This composition is remarkably constant.

Ricinoleic acid	89.5%
Dihydroxystearic acid	0.7%
Palmitic acid	1.0%
Stearic acid	1.0%
Oleic acid	3.0%
Linoleic acid	4.2%
Linolenic acid	0.3%
Eicosanoic acid	0.3%

The hydroxyl groups in castor oil account for a unique combination of physical properties: relatively high viscosity and specific gravity; solubility in absolute alcohol in any proportions; limited solubility in aliphatic petroleum solvents. The uniformity and reliability of its physical properties are demonstrated by the longtime use of castor oil as an absolute standard for viscosity tests. It has excellent emollient and lubricating properties.

The history of this substance in industry is in itself a long and fascinating story, too long to tell fully here. Briefly, however, it can be stated that because of the hydroxyl groups, double bonds, and ester linkages, which provide reaction sites, a number of chemical reactions in which castor oil is commercially used have been thoroughly explored. These include acetylation, alkoxylation, amination, caustic fusion, chemical dehydration, distillation, epoxidation, esterification, hydrogenation, oxidative polymerization, pyrolysis, and saponification. These reactions result in a multitude of oils, salts, glycerides, esters, amides, alcohols, halogens, and hydroxy-stearates.

Among the contributions of industry as it relates to the fields of medical inquiry and therapeutics is the work of A. F. Novak et al.,[24, 25] in using ricinoleic and oleic acid derivatives (both found in castor oil). These were screened for their antimicrobial activity, under optimum growing conditions, against several species of bacteria, yeasts, and molds. Several of the derivatives exhibited considerable inhibitory activity, comparable to sorbic and ten-undecenoic acid, known antimicrobial agents. Novak and his group stated that these substances warranted further study, since "the medicinal applications of some of these compounds might prove to be very important."

Industry played a large role in the work reported by Schwartz[26] in 1942, concerning the use of castor oil— among other constituents—in the make-up of protective ointments and cleansers. These were to be used where workers in industry would be subjected to exposure of irritating substances on the skin. His was an extensive report on the subject, and castor oil was found rather commonly in ointments and cleansers recommended.

From our own research at the A.R.E. Clinic,[27] the major findings included: (1) total lymphocyte count increased significantly in the group using castor oil packs; (2) T-pan lymphocyte count (T-11 cells) increased significantly in the group using castor oil packs, and the findings warranted further study of these packs on patients with chronic illness.

Our clinical experience with the castor oil packs applied over the abdomen led us to understand that the packs enhanced the function of the thymus gland and the other component parts of the immune system, making that system more effective in protecting the body from outside and inside dangers and helping the immune system take the lead in rebuilding any given part of the body. These findings, substantiated in early research, give this particular therapy an overall significance in laying the groundwork for a healing process to begin. The immune system is the foundation of health in the body, and it cannot be allowed to disintegrate or lose its normal abilities, or the body will be subject to illness in one area or another, depending upon where there are other weaknesses.

In line with these concepts, we have used the castor oil packs in every patient who has come to us for seizure problems (epilepsy). Cayce suggested that the packs would help rebuild and make more effective the Peyer's patches (patches of lymphoid tissue that are located in the walls of the small intestine), which are part of the immune system. According to these readings, these patches produce substances which are carried through the lymphatics and blood supply to the ailing portions of the nervous system that have caused the seizure problem in the first place.

In rendering these portions of the nervous system normal, Cayce suggested that the difficulty gradually can be eliminated. Always, however, he counseled that attitudes and emotional patterns need to be looked at and corrected or the changes will not come about.

Perhaps some of the understanding about how castor oil works can be found in the meditative experience. We seek in meditation to attune our physical and mental bodies to their Source, the divine energy we call God. The attunement has to be a vibrational exercise. When this is perfectly accomplished, illnesses of all sorts disappear. For in the God-Force, there is no illness.

The castor oil may create a vibration within the body that is more easily attuned to Creative Forces and thus bring a healing activity. We desperately need to find something other than medicines to bring healing to the body. This may be what alternative medicine is all about—the manner in which the vibrations of the human body can be attuned more effectively to the Divine and thus a healing appears, as if by magic. We call it a miracle. It may simply be an attunement! Cayce never saw it as a miracle. He described it as a spiritual event in this reading quoted earlier:

> Know that all strength, all healing of every nature is the changing of the vibrations from within—the attuning of the Divine within the living tissue of a body to Creative Energies. This alone is healing. Whether it is accomplished by the use of drugs, the knife or whatnot, it is the attuning of the atomic structure of the living cellular force to its spiritual heritage. (1967-1)

No matter what the cause, and even if we cannot yet comprehend how the effect is literally achieved, we do know that hyperactivity and a host of other conditions can be alleviated and most often eliminated through the simple act of applying a castor oil pack appropriately, consistently, and patiently to the body. And, through acts like that, the benefits of the castor bean plant demonstrate its right to the title it was given in the Middle ages: the Palma Christi, the palm of the Christ.

I recall that Cayce once said that there's as much of God in a teaspoonful of castor oil as there is in a prayer! That makes meditation, prayer, change of consciousness toward the Christ Consciousness, and material healing elements such as castor oil all one. Just as we are—at a deep level— one with the Creative Forces or God; as if we are truly— body, mind, and spirit—One. The human being is a wonderful creation—let's treat each other and ourselves that way, remembering that when God is at work in the healing process, anything good can happen.

Chapter Eight
Castor Oil in
Folk Medicine

MANY OF THE HABIT PATTERNS WHICH WE CALL our way of life come to us through the medium of verbal instruction, person to person. We see the constant use of this method in the home, school, and church. Yet a mother caring for her child is called "instinctive" as she applies wisdom which she had never been taught. As she kisses her child's finger where he or she has banged it on a board, she instinctively applies a healing touch. Throughout the history of humanity on the earth, much information in treating and caring for the body has been passed on through word of mouth and through that which has been called the unconscious mind.

Castor oil as a treatment for the body certainly has been a factor in the habit patterns of cultures throughout the past several thousand years, so it is not surprising to find the oil mentioned in the legends and stories of people and in folk medicine, wherever such practice exists in the world today.

From personal communications I found two stories about the use of castor oil which have their roots in folk history. After I had suggested some castor oil applications for her, Mrs. Carrie Hulsman told me in September 1965 that her old family doctor in Shelbyville, Indiana, always told her that "castor oil will leave the body in better condition than it found it."

In the Virginia mountains, midwives still deliver babies, and herb medicine still clears up conditions that the pharmacopoeia has left untouched. And the second story originates there. E. J. McCready told me in May 1965 of his visit some years ago to a Virginia mountain town where his sister lived. McCready had developed an intensely inflamed index finger. A local physician advised him to go to a larger city to have a surgeon work on it. He was about to leave at once, for the finger was very painful, when his sister influenced him to show the finger to "Aunt Minnie" who lived up in the hills and who was a midwife. As soon as she saw it, she told him to wrap a flannel cloth soaked in castor oil around the finger and leave it there.

He followed her advice and direction, and by morning most of the inflammation and all of the soreness were gone. By the morning of the second day, all the swelling and inflammation had gone and a grain of sand (acquired while he was bathing on the seashore one week earlier) was discovered under the edge of the fingernail. This came out with the castor oil bandage and the finger was healed.

D. C. Jarvis, in his book about the Vermont style of folk medicine,[28] listed many topical uses for castor oil. Among the more interesting are for warts anywhere on the body, for any kind of body ulcer, to heal the slow-to-heal umbilicus of a newborn infant, applied locally to breasts to increase flow of milk, for irritation of the conjunctivae of the eye, for lack of proper growth of hair in little children, and applied to eyelashes or eyebrows to stimulate growth.

He also included one for hunting dogs when they develop irritation of the eyes from running through the grass. The remedy: a few drops of castor oil.

Jarvis states in his book that aching feet can be made to feel much better and perform their duties more perfectly if, twice a week or more often, the feet are rubbed down at bedtime with castor oil. Then cotton socks should be slipped on and the oil left on overnight. In the morning, he states, the skin is like velvet, and generally all the tired, sore feeling will have disappeared. In the same way, castor oil can be used night and morning to soften corns and calluses and to remove the soreness. Castor oil is considered a specific remedy for corns.

In his experience, Jarvis found that castor oil would not only clear up warts, but also those skin afflictions known as papillomas of the skin, pigmented moles, and the more common "liver spots." The latter seem to come along with the aging process. According to Jarvis, the liver spots were not just improved, but were completely removed by some physiological process that left a clear skin without a sign of a blemish.

Chapter Nine
Castor Oil Working on the Body Physiology

EARLY IN MY USE OF CASTOR OIL PACKS in the practice of medicine, I had an interesting experience which taught me something about the real nature of the cells that go to make up this body of ours. I had been treating a woman for anemia. She had a hemoglobin of 9.3 grams (significantly below the norm). I had given her a product called Feosol, which supplies extra iron and was indicated for the anemia.

She returned six weeks later and I checked her hemoglobin again. It was still 9.3 grams. This time, however, she had a skin rash. It was not severe, but bothersome. Iron taken by mouth frequently causes a skin rash, and this was what appeared to be happening. I had read in the literature about a dermatologist who had given his patients castor oil by mouth which had cleared up the skin. So I suggested to this woman that she stop the iron and take an ounce of castor oil that night, repeat it in four days, and then let me see her again.

She didn't really hear me about the time factor, so she

70

showed up in another six weeks. She had felt so good that she kept on taking the castor oil every four days. I checked her skin. It was clear, of course. Her hemoglobin was next. Without the iron by mouth and with no other medication directed toward the anemia, her hemoglobin had risen to 13.4 and was normal.

What happened? Apparently the oil cleansed the cells that lined the upper intestinal tract where iron is absorbed from the food normally, and the body overcame its problem of iron deficiency. Cleansing, not iron tablets, healed the body.

It is a fascinating adventure to sift through the ideas and concepts found in the Edgar Cayce readings, and to sort out meaningful phrases and sentences which can lead one to a better understanding of the theory of the functioning of the human body as Cayce saw it while he was asleep.

Unfortunately, no one thought to ask him to give a consistent unconscious discourse on the subject of the human body when he was alive. And, during his waking hours, he was not privy to the information he tapped into while asleep.

It remains for us to play detective and to approach the comments which were made in the course of the readings with an open mind. We need to acknowledge that at our present state of understanding in the field of the healing arts, we may have approached ideas with a personal bias just as easily and with as much facility as our predecessors did a hundred or a thousand years ago.

WHAT HAPPENS TO THE PHYSIOLOGY WHEN CASTOR OIL IS USED ON THE HUMAN BODY?

Thus far, we have seen how Cayce's suggestions have been used to bring healing to the body in a variety of ways. Some of his readings give hints as to why this "oil that heals" brings about its responses. But we have not really investigated some of the bits of physiological activity that might be involved in that healing process.

An example of this is found in the instance of a forty-one-year-old man, who had difficulties which Cayce describe as uremic conditions. He was given the case number 2493-1, and it's a bit of a problem to give the man a clear medical diagnosis. Uremia does not coincide with the description in the reading of the man's condition, so we are left with a question in our minds. Cayce's description was that of a liver and kidney pathology which caused an unbalancing of the assimilating forces, and which did not appear to be of dire consequence, unlike uremia. In the doctor's office, the diagnosis would probably have been made of a vague gastrointestinal disorder.

In the readings, however, there is such a wide variety of disease syndrome present that it becomes evident that the castor oil packs were intended apparently to help in correcting conditions of disorder in the body that lie far beneath the surface. It is almost as if the entire autonomic nervous system is most often disturbed, creating in its abnormal activities a type of disturbed bodily function that we call a disease. This would give more understanding about the oil to the observer who sees a variety of disease processes respond to that same castor oil pack. This is a therapy, which, if it *does* affect the autonomic nervous system, is not really understood relative to the mechanics of its action.

Constipation has already been discussed to some extent. However, there have been some individuals who have requested a reading with this as one of the main complaints. The following excerpt illustrates how Cayce handled this problem:

> We find that the castor oil packs over the abdomen and right side would be well occasionally for the lack of eliminations. When these *are* applied, and the gen-

eral massage is given following same, give a quantity of olive oil—just so it is not sufficient to cause regurgitation or vomiting, we will find it will work well with the assimilating, and act as a food as well as an eliminant for the alimentary canal. (1553-7)

From the above, we are led to believe that Cayce would visualize a more healthy upper and lower gastrointestinal tract as a result of the use of the packs and the olive oil.

In another reading he was questioned at length by a young woman who wanted desperately to have a child and who thought at the time of the reading that she was pregnant. This, of course, involves the genitourinary system, another major functional area of the abdomen and pelvis. If the packs, as suggested in the above reading quoted, would bring ease to the stomach and bowels, we would assume—especially if the action *were* directed through the activity of the autonomic nervous system—that the generative organs, as well as the entire condition of pregnancy, would benefit from the same therapeutic administration. Reasons for this can best be described briefly as "proper balance" between the two components of the vegetative or autonomic nervous system: the sympathetic and the parasympathetic.

In the readings given for this woman who thought she was pregnant, much was disclosed about her fears and anxieties in the process of her present living. However, the part of the reading that becomes important is the following:

(Q) Would the continuing of castor oil packs for dissolving adhesions interfere with pregnancy—or tend to eliminate impregnation? Advise.

(A) Rather it would be advisable to use same, that when there is pregnancy it would prevent a great deal of distress and anxiety. (1523-12)

This reading tends to emphasize that the total effect on a pregnant woman would be similar to what we see today coming from the use of tranquilizers, although it would be expected that the side effects of the latter would not be encountered. Pregnancy, it would seem, would stand to benefit greatly from this kind of therapy. It becomes even more important to come to an understanding about just how the packs bring about their action.

The "how" might be given more clarity if we go back to the consideration of the lymphatics—the immune system—and have our question answered with another question, as we look at the following answer given to this person:

(Q) Condition of the lymphatic system?
(A) This is greatly improved, but there are still tendencies for the pockets to form, even in the end of the lymph ducts through the intestinal system. But with the continued use of the castor oil packs and the violet ray added, with the general treatment, it should be corrected. (2534-2)

It is sometimes difficult to understand exactly what Mr. Cayce meant in a reading. Here, it seems he is indicating that healing should come about with the suggested treatments, in the area that he describes as "the end of the lymph ducts through the intestinal system." It seems most logical to me to interpret that statement as pointing toward the very beginning of the lymph vessels, perhaps the villi of the small bowel where distention or pooling might most reasonably occur. These, at least, would be part of the "pockets" that Cayce describes.

It is known that the motor nerve supply of the lymphatics—the parasympathetic—is that which brings about peristalsis, so that pooling or distention does not occur.[29]

This raises the question of whether the packs applied on the abdomen influence the parasympathetic nerves to function more normally or whether their effect is directly on the immune system itself, the lymphatics in particular in this instance. Cayce leaves many of his statements unsupported, perhaps to encourage us to think them through or to do the research which establishes the mechanisms and the effects.

Another question that is raised is the balance or imbalance between the sympathetic and the parasympathetic nervous systems. Is the instance of the woman who thought she was pregnant one in which the sympathetic is too effective and too strong in its action so that it overpowers its counterpart, the parasympathetic? Many answers sometimes produce more questions, most of which at the present time remain unanswered.

The wide variety of problems presented for solution through Cayce's psychic readings is exemplified by case 5146-1, a minister's wife who sought help to relieve symptoms from a series of traumatic events in her life. At the time of the reading she had been troubled by "bladder weakness," which was aggravated by sexual intercourse. Against the background of much worry in the church situation where her husband ministered, she found mice in her davenport, picked them up, wriggling in her hand, and suffered extreme psychologic trauma which brought about a painful bladder distention.

Shortly afterward, she was bitten by a dog, developed upset stomach, then a urinary frequency that necessitated her voiding every twenty-five minutes. This was followed by such a fear of voiding unconsciously that she found herself unable to attend any church service or social function. Finally, she developed a vocal disturbance which rendered her unable to sing.

In years past, doctors may not have found any physical

problem in this case and would have told her it was in her mind. In the middle years of this century, it would have been called a psychosomatic illness. Today I view such a situation as emotional disturbances and life situations creating a complex set of neurological imbalances that, in turn, resulted in physical and physiological illness. Somewhere in the vegetative or autonomic nervous system there certainly would be located a variety of disturbed impulses.

In this case, Cayce suggested first a series of the castor oil packs associated with the administration of olive oil. He added another type of pack, also suggested osteopathic manipulations, and gave the woman considerable dietary advice about refraining from sweets and pastries. The comment found in his answer to the first question after the main body of the reading, however, contains information which is interesting in the light of comments above concerning the autonomic nervous system:

> This treatment, as we find, will aid in the body's gaining better control of all activities of the sympathetic [vegetating] nervous system. For those taxations, through the poisons as well as the actual pain through [the] alimentary canal, have been the sources, and the acidity through the system. This will help in these directions. (5146-1)

Cayce's suggestions seem to be aimed at bringing about a relaxation of the tensions found in the autonomic nervous systems, or perhaps a better balance between the two parts of it—all through physically applied therapies. No record is available of the results, since the woman apparently did not follow through on the therapy program suggested. Or at least she did not share her experiences with Mr. Cayce.

MIGRAINE HEADACHES
AND OTHER PHYSIOLOGICAL PROBLEMS

Always associated with significant tensions, migraines create rather exquisite pain and disturbance, and have been, in medical history, chronically unresponsive to therapy. This condition is anatomically as far removed from the bladder as possible, yet Cayce finds a relationship in the etiology of the headaches and the bladder problem just discussed. This helps us to realize that the entire body is one unit, no matter how far apart the symptoms may appear anatomically.

A man, thirty years old, had experienced severe headaches, diagnosed as migraine, since he was fourteen years old. All attempts at therapy had been failures. To Cayce, the cause and cure of this condition were relatively simple; his discussion lengthy, yet fascinating:

These as we find arise from a condition that exists through the alimentary canal, especially as part of the circulation in the colon. From the pressure there arises the periodic headaches that are the source of the general nervous disturbance in the body.

These as we find may be removed. They are the sources of those that are at times called the types of headaches which refuse to respond to any of the ordinary treatments, and will become constitutional unless there is something done about it.

As we find we would have the application once or twice a week of castor oil packs. If these could be given regularly for several days, it might be more easily eliminated. But when it is practical, at least twice a week, apply over the abdomen, and especially the caecum, and extending up the right side to the gall duct area, castor oil packs. Keep them on for at least one hour or one and one-half hours at the time. Cover this with an electric pad when it has been covered so that it doesn't soil the linens from the oil. Make the pack with two or three thicknesses of flannel, preferably old flannel; saturate the flannel, not just pour on, but saturate the flannel with the castor oil.

The next day take internally at least 2 tablespoons of olive oil.

Each time following the application of the oil packs, massage the body along the spine, especially the areas from the lumbar axis to that area between the shoulders, with cocoa butter; massage this thoroughly for at least fifteen to twenty minutes, and let all the cocoa butter that the body will absorb be rubbed into same.

This, as we find, if it is followed, will relieve the sources of this disturbance . . .

(Q) Is this connected with the foot trouble which has recently developed, and what causes this?

(A) This is, as has been indicated, a part of the condition. Massage from the lumbar axis. Foot trouble is a reflex pressure on the nerves that lead to the brain through the nerves of the sympathetic system to the cerebrospinal center. (5052-1)

This patient followed the suggestions which were given, rather rapidly improved, and later reported that he was completely free of the condition.

In this instance of the man with the migraine headaches and the minister's wife with her traumatic experiences, the autonomic nervous system is involved directly, as seen from Cayce's psychic perspective. It becomes more and more obvious that there is difficulty in discussing etiology and therapy, as Cayce "saw" things without considering the most basic physiological functionings of the various organs and systems of the body and their associated control by the vegetative (autonomic) nervous system impulses and control. Cayce refers to this kind of control, often discussing it at length, in many of the physical readings.

The parents of a two-and-a-half-year-old girl applied for a reading because their daughter was anemic and not growing as vigorously as she should. In the second reading she was given, it became apparent that she had vaginitis, and the question and answer dealing with this problem is worthy of being quoted:

(Q) What causes the irritated condition, seemingly in the vaginal passage, and what should be done for it?
(A) Use packs of castor oil across the lower portion of the abdomen and the lacteal duct, for about an hour twice a week for two to three weeks; and this then, with the rest of the rubs, should make for an alleviation. This tendency for irritation is from the *acidity* in the system. (785-2)

The castor oil, in this instance, is suggested to be used across the abdomen over the "lacteal duct" to control a vaginal irritation in a child. Similar therapy has been suggested through the readings for uterine fibroids and pelvic conditions of all sorts, including what is listed as pelvic cellulitis.

This particular reading extract, because of its simplicity, tells us several things about the manner of action of the packs in pelvic conditions, as well as indicating something about the causation of at least some of these cases. Cayce saw an *acidity* in the body. It is known that vaginitis is in most cases associated with an excess local alkalinity. The blood and body cells tend to keep a constant pH (hydrogen ion concentration) in the body as a whole.

It may be here that abnormal physiological functioning brings about an overall acidity through the body excreting more substances of an alkaline nature. The alkalinity of the vaginal tract may be synonymous with disease, while the acidity of those tissues brings about health. The question of acid-alkaline balance in the body and the effect it has on health is difficult to answer simply, if at all. For there appears to be an overall need to keep the bloodstream and the body tissue cells at location-specific pH levels for health to be obtained. The lymphatic system, for instance, is at a higher pH norm than the bloodstream. And each group of cells/organs/systems seems to know what level spells health or disease for it.

In regard to the mode of action in at least some cases of pelvic pathology, we might assume that one of several things would come about to bring these areas into better health. The packs, when applied over the abdomen, could create an effect within the autonomic nerve supply to the pelvis, either changing the tissue reaction and bringing about a more acid pH to the secretions or, through the nerve impulses to the tissues, influencing the lymphatic drainage for the better in a direct manner or via the autonomic. Also the packs could bring about a more adequate drainage of the metabolic protein wastes of the cells from the intercellular spaces, thus leaving the cells more healthy. These theoretical considerations seem to be implied in these readings, as seemingly unconnected comments are gradually brought into focus.

In one of the earliest cases in which castor oil packs were advised, a seventy-five-year-old woman (15-2) was being treated by her physicians for what was diagnosed as a cancer of the abdominal cavity, causing obstruction which was almost complete. The woman was nauseated and vomited constantly despite all efforts. Bowel contents were brought up every time. Cayce's reading stated that this was not a cancer, but fecal impaction and tissue swelling which could be alleviated. She was given three readings, but there is unfortunately no record of what happened subsequent to that.

Thus we have neither a final diagnosis nor even an indication of how diligently the application of the various suggestions was carried out.

It becomes obvious that Cayce's internal "perception" of the human body led him to make observations while asleep that were at variance with accepted medical ideas of that day and this. The fascinating aspect of his perception, however, is the consistency of results obtained from his suggestions, based on his understanding of the pathology plus the remarkable internal consistency of his comments regarding what was happening to the body physiology in such a wide variety of cases. There seems to be a continuing basic functioning according to certain (what he would consider) universal rules, and this basic functioning appears to be what he describes case after case.

From the time when immunizations were first begun, there have been individuals who have vigorously objected to the procedure for a variety of reasons. In the early years of the use of smallpox vaccination, the procedure was condemned by a gradually decreasing number of physicians. Today, there are still those who feel that these procedures, in spite of their preventive values, have a detrimental effect on the tissues of the body in certain instances.

The reading that follows addresses certain physical changes that came about as a result of immunizations given earlier. For obvious reasons, these psychic statements have led and will lead to disagreement and perhaps controversy. However, while asleep, Cayce in his readings seemed to cut across the boundaries of opinion in the total field of healing, drawing from many sources, and claiming that no single concept of healing today is wholly right or sacrosanct. This is not a popular stand to take, but this is Cayce throughout his readings.

The lacteals come into more evaluation in the next quote from the readings. A thirteen-year-old boy was described as having difficulty of the lacteals. Physiology texts describe them as those areas within the villi of the small intestine which initiate the absorption of fat from the intestinal tract, the digestive portion of what we call assimilation of foods. This is a portion of the reading:

> Now, as we find, there are very definite disturbances in the physical forces of this body.
> As we find, these have arisen from properties as were injected for preventions in the physical reactions of the body. Hence those portions of the body have become involved from which assimilations produce those elements necessary for the replenishing of organs, of activity, of all forces of the body.
> Thus the lacteal ducts are involved, or those portions where first the digestive forces draw from the digestion that influx of activity for the body.
> So the whole of the left portion of the body is involved, but affectation arises from the right portion or caecum area.
> Not the affectation of the vermiform appendage but rather that from which such conditions may arise eventually, without correction; yet involving more the lacteal area and the gall duct and the glandular system.
> From same then very poor digestion arises at times, also a low blood pressure, a very slow pulsation and a general anemia.
> These as we find are those disturbing forces in this body.
> As we find, then, in making applications of those things that may be helpful, we must take into consideration all portions of the system involved and build to that as will stimulate the activity for a more perfect balance; and allow the system through its coordination to adjust the conditions. (1123-2)

How would the lacteal ducts become involved? Would this lack of proper absorption bring about all the other changes described? These are questions that cannot be answered at this time. From this reading, however, is seen another facet of Cayce's philosophy which undergirds most of the information found here, and which will be part of this book throughout: to "allow the system through its coordination to adjust the conditions." Cayce instructs the individual, after balance is brought more perfectly to the body, to do just this. This implies that there is a force of life which flows through the body at all times that will be a healing force, *if* balance is such that it can flow adequately. Cayce apparently sees balance and coordination as being actual physical forces within the body which can be affected through administration of different types of healing instrumentalities. These he sees as being medications, massages, packs, exercises, inhalations, breathing adjustments, cleansing (colonics, etc.), and attitudes of the mind, emotions, and spirit.

MORE PHYSIOLOGY

In a number of his readings, Cayce suggested olive oil to be taken following the use of the castor oil packs. Let's see why he used both the packs and olive oil. It is well known that fat or oil taken into the stomach causes the gall bladder and the large bile ducts to contract through the action of a hormone known as cholecystokinin,[30] released from the walls of the stomach into the bloodstream.

Olive oil would produce an increase in the flow of bile both from the liver and the gall bladder, which in turn would act as a catharsis and stimulate even further increased flow of bile.

This following extract from the readings implies such physiological activity:

(Q) How long should the castor oil pack be kept up and how often?
(A) Keep up the packs until the corrections and the lesions in the area are broken up. These should be taken by periods, three days at a time, an hour each day. Follow same with two teaspoonfuls of olive oil. We wish to clear the alimentary canal and keep it clear . . . Leave off these packs after three days for two weeks and then give them again. (5379-1)

The next extract, however, indicates that the combination of the packs, the oil, and a heating pad also bring about activity within the body that is obviously what was desired.

Apply castor oil packs over the liver area about one hour each day for two days, then give internally two teaspoonfuls of olive oil after the second day. Apply the castor oil pack with at least three thicknesses of flannel, saturated with the castor oil, and then apply the electric pad over same. This should stir the liver into activity. These are what is needed to remove the tendency for strep. (2299-12)

A sixty-three-year-old woman (reading 3683-1) was told that her difficulty was in large part caused by a malfunction of the liver. In Cayce's terminology, she was told that the right lobe of the liver was causing distresses to the pancreas and the spleen, while the liver as a whole was causing distresses to the kidneys and bladder, the lung, heart, and the assimilating system.

This comment underscores one of the most important, yet medically unrecognized, physiological activities that occurs in the human body. If a malfunctioning liver can distress the kidney, for instance, there must be a coordination that normally exists between the two organs. Neither operates in a vacuum. In reality, none of the organs or systems works by itself. If these portions of the body have consciousness, then there must be a cooperation or a coordination among all of them in order to have health as a portion of that person's experience.

"Let's all cooperate!" they seem to be saying to each other. But emotional impact, through the medium of the endocrine system, seems so often to thwart this effort toward cooperation. An example would be when an ulcer is formed because a man's boss really hates him, then cooperation and coordination are lost and illness sets in.

In the reading cited above, recommended treatment consisted of castor oil packs before anything else. This would indicate that Cayce, in his unconscious state, "saw" the necessity of improving the conditions of the liver before anything else would or, perhaps, could be done. This implies that one of the functions of the castor oil packs is an enhancement of the liver function, not only in its ability to be the detoxifier of the body, but also in its beneficial effect to all the surrounding organs rather than being a dross and a distress to them. Cayce implies that when the liver is not functioning normally, it can and often does act as an irritant to some or all of the organs in any way relating to the liver in their activity.

There is specific information on this particular circumstance that is either missing or as yet undiscovered in the readings. We do know, however, that the liver produces one-third to one-half of all the lymph produced in the human body under resting conditions. This, along with the lymph from the intestines, constitutes half of all that is produced in the body.[31]

This might shed some light on the importance of the liver in body physiology. The lymph plays an enormous role, however, along with the liver, in affecting the health of the body. And it is a fascinating liquid.

For instance, the lymph from the liver contains six grams percent protein concentration, just a bit less than that of normal plasma in the bloodstream. From most areas of the body, lymph has a protein concentration of only one-and-a-half percent. Thus, when these are mixed as they are in the thoracic duct and then into the venous system of the body, the concentration of protein is about three to four percent.

The lymph also has considerable fat in it, arising from the villi of the small intestines. These normal structures of the small bowel have central lymphatic capillaries called central lacteals. After a fatty meal, thoracic-duct lymph resembling milk in its appearance, sometimes contains as high as one or two percent fat. The lymphatic system is one of the major channels of absorption from the gastrointestinal tract, being principally responsible for the absorption of fats. This absorbed material then passes upward through the thoracic duct to enter the bloodstream.[32] Lymphatic vessels of the intestinal canal are called lacteals because of this appearance and function.

The lymphatics are indeed a unique portion of the circulation of the body. They not only drain the villi in the intestinal tract, they also have other beginnings in all distant parts of the body. Lymph flows in only one direction, gathering its substance, like a mountain stream, in tiny rivulets.

The lymph has its origins in the intercellular spaces throughout the body and in the central lacteals of the small intestine. As the lymph vessels grow larger and larger, they coalesce and finally empty into collecting vessels, the right lymphatic and the thoracic duct, and then on into the right and left subclavian veins; thence into the largest vein of the body, the vena cava. From there, the lymph becomes part of the blood as it is pumped by the heart through the lungs and then into the general circulation, as arterial, oxygen-bearing liquid.

From the foregoing, the lymph would seem to have at least two functions—one associated with the lacteals and the absorption and assimilation of foods and the other as a cleansing or drainage system of the cells. In this manner, the lymphatics would constitute the first stage of eliminations which must occur in the body in order to keep the body healthy.

The lacteals were mentioned frequently in the Cayce readings. It was inevitable that someone would ask the direct question about their identity from Cayce's unconscious mind. This was his answer:

That portion that makes for the ability of the system to take from the food values and prepare same in the manner in which same may be used to revivify, revitalize, recharge the system itself. (1055-1)

Cayce's explanation, then, might be that the term *lacteals* would include all those structures which take part in the assimilation of food from the intestines and its preparation in the process so that it could be taken via the bloodstream to nourish the tissues of the body. This would include the villi themselves, the lymph, the single lymph nodules, and the Peyer's patches found in the wall of the small bowel. It would also include the collecting lymphatics and the lymph nodes found along the way, through which the lymph passes.

The villi are those highly vascular structures which project from the mucous membrane into the lumen (cavity) of the small intestine throughout its entire length, and give to the surface of the intestine a velvety appearance. These villi are largest and most numerous in the duodenum, which is the first part of the small bowel, and in the jejunum, the second part. They become smaller and fewer in number in the ileum, the third part of the small bowel or intestine. There are none in the large bowel. They are placed remarkably close together and are so numerous that the surface area of the small intestine—one-half square meter normally—is increased to about ten square meters by means of these projections, covering nearly the entire surface of the small bowel.[33]

The individual villus is made up of a central lacteal, sometimes two, which is surrounded by retiform lymphoid tissue in which lie blood vessels and the longitudinal and circular muscular fibers; then surrounding these is found the basement membrane on which are placed the columnar and globular epithelial cells. These latter come into direct contact with the food as it passes down the lumen of the small bowel, and all absorption must come about here.

Peyer's patches are mentioned frequently in the readings. These lymphatic patches were discovered and described by Johann Conrad Peyer, a Swiss naturalist and anatomist in 1677. It is interesting that over 300 years have produced so little information about their function, but recently it has been shown that they are important in producing immunity to substances taken through the intestinal tract in the early years of life. And they are now known to be part of the immune system, which is generally understood these days to be directed by the thymus gland, located in the mediastinum of the chest, that area between the right and left lungs, where the heart is also found.

These patches are more correctly called aggregated lymphatic nodules[34]; but are also known as Peyer's glands, agminated follicles, or tonsillae intestinales. They form circular or oval patches, varying in length from two to ten centimeters, and the twenty to thirty patches which occur are found to be the largest and the most numerous in the ileum. While they are only occasionally observed in the duodenum, they are seen more frequently in the jejunum, but they are small and circular there. They are placed lengthwise in the intestine, and are situated in the portion of the tube which is most distant from the mesenteric attachment.

Each patch is formed of a group of solitary lymphatic nodules covered with mucous membrane, but the patches do not, as a rule, possess villae on their free surfaces. Anatomical observation has shown that they are best marked in the young person, they become indistinct in middle age, and sometimes disappear altogether in advanced life. They are given an abundant supply of blood from the plexus which surrounds each follicle. Vessels give off fine branches which permeate the lymphoid tissue in the interior of the follicles. The lymphatic plexuses are especially abundant around these patches.

The Cayce readings regard Peyer's patches as important portions of the body which have a great deal to do with longevity or the maintaining of full and abundant health. As I understand the readings that have something to do with health as a whole and especially in reference to these patches, it appears to me that Cayce was explaining that the health of the nervous system was, to an extent, maintained through the substances that the Peyer's patches elaborate when they—the patches—are in good health. Cayce touched on this in the following reading:

> Now, in the physical forces of the body (as seen and understood, in the nervous systems of the body), there are those glands that secrete fluids which in the circulation sustain and maintain the reaction fluid in the nerve channels themselves. (271-5)

Apparently, the substance produced by these patches is, under normal circumstances, made a part of the lymphocytes formed there and is then carried through the bloodstream to the areas where electrical contact is made between the autonomic and the cerebrospinal nervous system. This relationship and the need for it to remain normal and balanced have an important role to play in the causation and/or correction of seizure disorders, more commonly called epilepsy.

The role of these patches is touched on in the last reading that Cayce ever gave, which was for himself and his rather desperate condition late in 1944. These patches described by Johann Peyer were called in this reading as "those patches that are called by a man's name." Sometimes, it is important, in studying the readings, to be a good detective. Here is the reading:

> For the excess use of salines to flush or to cleanse the colon has reduced in blood more of that which causes that plasm. Thus the inabilities of those centers, those patches through which there are the areas of the lymph circulation, are such as to cause ofttimes a state of disintegration. In these patches, then, there is a lack of sufficient globular forces to cause the coagulation in the flow of the lymph, or that portion of same which is the leucocyte, or the sticky portion in the blood is not sufficient to make perfect contact between sympathetic and cerebrospinal activities of the body.
>
> Those congestions caused in the trachea, the conditions in the heart activity—the pressure is near normal at most times. When there is overexercise physically, or especially the mental forces as of worry or anxiety, to be sure it calls on the necessity of these emunctory activities—or those patches that are called by a man's name. These are then lessened in their number and thus make a quickening, or an anxiety, causing the flow of blood in the heart, as an organ, to dilate . . .

In making administrations to supply these glandular centers which supply to these patches, or the
emunctories add these in the B complex or the ribo-
flavin—the necessary elements in each portion of the
B vitamin forces. (294-212)

Perfect contact between the sympathetic and cerebrospinal nervous systems, made possible through
substances created in these small patches of lymphatic tissue in the mucosal surface of the small intestine—a concept
which is indeed exciting—leads us to wonder just what part
these patches play in the physical disturbances that come
about when we are subjected to stresses and worries that
we hold on to in our minds and the emotional parts of our
bodies.

Cayce's ability to pinpoint problem areas is still not well
understood, even by those who study his readings. In reading number 4595-1, he described a leakage of lymph from
the fourth left dorsal sympathetic ganglion into the blood
circulation. This leakage came into being because of a lack
of the coagulating forces which Cayce saw as being normally formed in the lymphatic system. This, in turn, caused
the arterial vessel walls to produce a substance which is carried throughout the body, disturbing the function of all the
organs. He suggested therapy for a period of forty-eight
days, which he described as being a cycle of relationship
between the sympathetic and cerebrospinal nervous systems.

These are strange to us—these new functions brought
into focus in the lymphatics and their subsequent relationship to the nervous system. The next reading extract leads
us to understand that the globular substance which the
patches apparently manufacture has been increased and is
bringing into being a repair in the nerve contacts by means
of formation of a filamentous substance:

There is still at times incoordination in the
sympathetics through the activities to the cerebrospinal and to the sensory reactions (we are speaking from
the physical angle entirely in the present, you see), yet
there has been created—by the activities of the properties in the system—more of a stimuli to the
coordinating reactions, in the form of filaments of circulation through the activities of plasm in the nerve
forces themselves, as well as a better application of the
blood supply about those portions through which the
nerve plasm operates. (386-3)

The ideas in the Cayce material regarding the lymphatics
and their functions, not usually considered in approaching
the body physiology, are certainly worth considering when
attempting to understand how the body works. Such consideration is especially important for the ideas that apply to
the understanding of the use of castor oil packs on the human body.

Some years ago several studies were reported on the flow
of lymph in problems involving the lungs and the heart.[35]
One experiment involved venting of the thoracic duct in
nine patients who were in the final stages of heart disease
and had huge thoracic ducts distended with lymph under
pressure. Within twenty-four hours, central venous pressures fell toward normal. Distended neck veins, peripheral
edema, ascites, and liver tenderness all diminished or disappeared. Liver edges disappeared under the costal
margins.

An enormous excess of lymph is formed in patients with
Laënnec's cirrhosis. Dr. Dumont pointed out that vessels
designed to carry off this fluid become widely distended
and incompetent. When the distended thoracic duct is
vented, ascites disappears, portal vein pressure drops, and
liver size decreases.

We have seen how individuals have applied castor oil packs over various parts of their bodies and the lymphatic system responds to the castor oil and brings healing to the body. In the findings reported above, we might find some of the essential functions of the lymph at work or failing to work.

When we consider the cannulation of the thoracic duct and its results, we see that this procedure is a removal of the lymph with its contents from its normal flow to be taken from the body entirely. The lymph, you will recall, is the first stage of elimination from the cells of the body. This venting of the lymph produces a marked improvement in the condition of the body. The lymphatics, through the venting procedure, is a cleansing of the lymph and the bloodstream.

Body wastes, substances which are the result of cellular metabolism and extruded from the cell, must be removed through the lymph. In this procedure, no matter how unusual it may be, the cleansing is performed and the body, as a result, is allowed to become more normal. Waste products are taken out of the body instead of being allowed to stay within the circulating bloodstream, where they would have to be removed by the body's organs of excretion—the kidneys, the lungs, liver and intestines, and the skin.

If such a procedure brings about a return to a more normal central venous pressure in a patient with advanced heart failure and if the distended neck veins disappear—if in reality the peripheral edema, the ascites, the liver tenderness, and liver engorgement all disappear or regress markedly—then this would seem to indicate that this sick body needs one thing in particular: proper elimination of the substances which are found in the lymphatic fluid, which in this case are being vented to the outside.

If this fluid or its contents, which represent in one sense a washing of the individual cells of the body, could be purified and the products of metabolism eliminated from the body other than by cannulation, then it is not only feasible, but understandable, that the body itself, under proper conditions, could return all these pathological findings to as normal a condition *without* the cannulation.

Such a return to normal would be predicated on changing the functioning of the organs of elimination at their cellular level in such a way that the waste products carried by the lymph would be eliminated normally from the body rather than being retained.

Cayce defines all portions of the body as being vital to the rest, and at times describes activities and relationships in a rather sweeping manner. Another excerpt from reading 5379-1 relates the coccyx, the lacteal duct in the area of the umbilicus, and the nervous system with special reference to the medulla oblongata to the seizures associated with the spasmodic reactions found in epilepsy:

> Now, as we find, there are disturbances in the developments of this body. In some time back there was an injury to the end of the spine so that the coccyx end of the spine is turned in to the side and this causes the conditions which develop in the right side, especially in the area of the umbilical and lacteal duct, and these at certain periods will increase unless corrected because the spasmodic reaction is the medulla oblongata, the larger nerve center in the base of the brain, which causes contractions and spasmodic reactions. (5379-1)

These relationships are somewhat like the physical changes and functional improvements that happened to a woman in one of our residential programs. We call these the Temple Beautiful Programs, named originally in 1978, when we started working with people in a residential setting. As mentioned in Chapter Six, the programs were named after the Temple Beautiful which Cayce said started more than

10,000 years ago in ancient Egypt. Also, the name was chosen because we knew that each individual is really the temple of the living God, and there He has promised to meet us. So each person attending is himself or herself the Temple Beautiful. It has certainly turned out that way.

The woman I referred to in the last paragraph told me on the phone before the program began that her physicians had found stones in both kidneys. One kidney had no function whatsoever, the other only twenty percent. She didn't know if she would be able to make the plane trip. Subsequently she fainted three times while in the plane. She was told that she would eventually need a kidney transplant.

She had passed kidney stones many times and her outlook was indeed bleak from the conventional point of view. However, one of the concepts we have gained from the Cayce readings is that there are no conditions that cannot be returned to normal health. Perhaps we don't always have the formula for this kind of result, but it is possible.

What happened over those days in the Temple Beautiful Program was remarkable. The day after she arrived, she was out in the spacious lawn of the Oak House, moving and dancing with the colored sheets to the beautiful music of the classics (plus a little polka) and the yellow color of her face began to clear up.

By the last day of the program, she was vital-looking, beautiful, and enthusiastic about the future. The diet, the dreams, castor oil packs, group sessions, electromagnetic therapy, massages and colonics, and counseling had played their part in a healing process that bears much promise for her through the days and years ahead. She truly has an opportunity to regenerate the kidneys and live a happy, healthy life.

Healing of the human body is dealt with in many ways in the Cayce readings. The following are some explanations that speak directly to the results just reported on:

For, in each physical body (and with this body, [257]), there are the abilities for the body to revive, resuscitate, reorganize itself continuously. It is only the consciousness that the activities of the body wastes with age, care, fear, doubt or the like, that produces what ye term old age or decrepitness in the activities of the body physically and mentally. (257-191)

As indicated, all the elements for revivifying, or for producing reproduction of functionings of organs, functionings of activities, functionings of nerve forces, are produced by glands. (360-4)

It is always helpful to remember that, after resuscitation and balance are brought more perfectly to the body, we need to allow the system through its coordination to adjust the condition. This implies that there is a force of life which flows through the body at all times that will be a healing force when the body's balance is such that it can flow adequately. Cayce apparently sees balance and coordination as being actual physical forces within the body which can be affected through administration of different types of healing instrumentalities, such as massages, castor oil packs, exercises, inhalations, breathing adjustments, medications, surgery, and the attitudes of mind, emotions, and spirit.

We must remember that attitudes, emotions, and beliefs all have their part in determining the health and constructive activity of the glandular structures of the body. This is the likely connection among thoughts and emotions, the functioning of the organs and systems, and the health or lack of it of the body.

Chapter Ten
Attitudes and
Emotions in Healing

ATTITUDES AND EMOTIONS PLAY A PART IN ALL healing experiences. Faith in the therapy, in the therapist, or in the God Force is an attitude, strengthened by repetitive activity. It is well known that such faith, even though it might not be the greatest in the world, aids in healing the body.

Many years ago I suggested to a fifty-eight-year-old woman that she use a castor oil pack on her abdomen to ease the discomfort she developed from an episode of vomiting. She had never heard of such treatment before, but she readily agreed to use it according to the directions I gave her.

When I saw her three days later, she was feeling great. "That pack was the best tranquilizer I have ever used!" she exclaimed. Maybe it was the activity of the pack itself that did the relaxing and the healing, but it was aided by her attitude of acceptance of and trust in me as her physician.

One cannot go through the physical readings and fail to come to the conclusion that emotions and attitudes of mind play a great part in the illnesses that have to do with portions of the body treated with castor oil packs. The psyche and the soma seemed at times to be one, as far as the Cayce readings are concerned. A good example is the instance of this woman who had gall bladder disease:

> Much might be said about the attitude the body has held that has caused a great deal of, or been a contributing cause to, the great distresses [cholecystitis] that come to the body; especially in the extremities, as these have grown to be in tendons, as the body has held resentments in the body... Eliminating these will be getting only partially at the seat of the trouble. (3196-1)

How does an attitude affect the physical body? How would it create an illness in the body? Why did Edgar Cayce say that a thought is a thing? These are questions that have puzzled searchers many years. I have thought of a "thing" as something that one could pick up and handle, like a tool, or a piece of bread, or a steering wheel. But one cannot pick up or handle a thought. And an attitude in a real sense is a thought.

Cayce had no problem with this concept:

> To be sure, attitudes oft influence the physical conditions of the body. No one can hate his neighbor and not have stomach or liver trouble. (4021-1)

In the spiritual realm, we understand God as bringing material things into reality, while creating us as counterparts of Himself. Such an understanding still doesn't answer the question about how an attitude can bring about changes in a physical body. What physiology is involved?

Perhaps it is most simply explained by acknowledging that emotions are basically located in the endocrine glands. These glands send nerve impulses throughout the body and, at the same time, produce and distribute hormones in accord with the kind of emotions being engendered. The chemicals thus produced are potent and direct activities in the autonomic nervous system and in various functioning organs. These chemicals produce conditions that we know as hypertension, ulcer of the stomach, heart disease, and a host of other illnesses that have not yet been recognized as having their origin in what we decide to think or to "feel."

Our emotions create either constructive or destructive habit patterns in the glands, as we use these emotions repeatedly over a period of time. The glands "do their thing," in a sense, to the autonomic nervous system. Then the physiology as a whole responds to create a physical illness that is a mirror image of the kind of thought that has been created as a pattern or habit in the mind of the glands.

It may help to look at how a karmic influence—a memory from past lifetimes, and thus a thought imbedded in the consciousness—was seen by Edgar Cayce to create a paralysis in the body of a thirty-nine-year-old man. We can say that the karma affected the nervous system, perhaps through the circulation or through the influences of the endocrine glands—in this case, the adrenals, where power and forgiveness lie side by side:

> Before this, then, the entity was in the land of the present sojourn, in those associations with the activities in the struggle for freedom on the part of some with whom the entity joined; yet the mercilessness of the savage (as would be termed in the present) was indicated in the orders given by the entity in dealing with characters and activities.

And these rendered many helpless. Ye are meeting
same in thine own self. And some of those upon whom
ye meted those measures must today measure to thee
in patience.

Thus gain *ye* in that experience, through knowing
that as ye sow, that must ye reap. For, life—the manifestation of that power, that influence ye call God—is
continuous; and self must be purged that ye may walk
as one with Him.

For whom He loveth He chasteneth. Love *thou* thy
fellow man! Manifest that ye would have measured to
thee in thy daily life . . .

So live today, then, that life that ye may look *every*
one in the face and say, "The Lord forgive thee, as I forgive thee." (2564-3)

This man was living under the influence of thoughts he
had chosen to make real because of his activities in a past
life. They created a pattern. The pattern then brought about
a condition of his physical body through the workings of
the unconscious mind. All the time, I'm sure, he was asking
himself and probably others, "Why did this happen to me?"

His answer might have been found in another Cayce
statement. This man apparently acted in error, a wrong direction according to his soul purpose in the earth. Cayce
reminds all of us:

For God alone quickens into life that which has
through any form of error misdirected its flow through
even the physical body. (1152-5)

It's a wonderful manner in which we are made. We have
been told over and over again by the Cayce readings that
the power of choice is God's greatest gift to us and we must
learn to treasure that heritage and use it, not abuse it. In

that way, we can create a new being!

In his readings, Cayce seemed to sense the relationship of each part of the body to another portion, so that function then became a total working together. A weakening of one portion of the body often produced trouble and distress throughout the entire body. Cayce warned one man in his use of the packs:

> We would make these material applications. Don't do it until you have prayed very oft, or it'll be more harm than good! (3492-1)

This suggestion is stranger than psychosomatic direction because it has spiritual overtones, which Cayce seemed to find necessary in his explanation of the nature of the body. From the same reading, comes the following:

> Do this [the packs] for at least three series, after you have found yourself and your relationships to the Creator. Without finding that, apply it not. (3492-1)

An unusual set of directions for application of the packs is also given in the same reading. The directions imply that the packs, when applied, can send a radiation of cleansing activity throughout the entire body. The mechanism is not described, only the mention that this will happen:

> Apply the packs warm, sufficient to make for that radiation of activity to the body, and then apply the electric pad—that throughout the whole body there may be that radiation which brings the elimination of poisons from the body (3492-1)

This reading brings us back to the considerations which already have been touched upon—those dealing with eliminations, even from the cells themselves. Cayce's "radiation" might be an effect brought on through the autonomic nervous system. It also could be an electromagnetic radiation, because electricity is seen in the readings as the manifestation of the Divine—not God, but the *manifestation* of God. We each must remember that we are all electrical organisms, since each body is composed of atoms and all atoms are electrical units.

Being an electrical being, we are an energy being and we probably will go further in understanding ourselves and others as we see our emotions and our attitudes affecting our bodies at an energy level, deriving the results often from past-life experiences.

One of Cayce's readings deals with cause and correction of a problem, not from the standard medical viewpoint, but from the perspective which Cayce used to see the human as an eternal being, creative in nature and one with the Creative Forces, yet in essence subject to building health or disease in the physical body, depending on what that one has done with one's mind and choices.

Cayce in this following reading was talking about the conflict between spirit and flesh as causing illness, and he was referring to two whom Jesus had healed:

What has ever been the builder, body, mind and spirit? As given, the expressions are in the physical, the motivative force is the spirit, the mind is the builder. What was builded? Those bodies had dwelt as individuals do (as may be illustrated in habit) with the interconsciousness of the necessity of the expression of something within self which brought dis-ease, the natural result of what? An at-variance to the divine law! Hence it may truly be said that to be at-variance may bring sickness, dis-ease, disruption, distress in a physical body. It is true then that the mind may heal entirely by the spoken word, by the laying on of hands, dependent upon the *consciousness* of the motivative forces in the individual body. Yet those requiring material expression to create a balance may necessitate drug, knife, water, heat, electricity, or *any* of those forces that are yet what? What is the spirit? The *manifestation of God!* The *Creative* Force working in, with and upon what? The awareness, the interconsciousness of the *body,* the mind, the spirit, as separated in individuals! (262-83)

Stresses, strains, and tensions become part of everyone's experience and often create the disruptions and distresses in the physical body that Cayce talked about. They always play a role in the pH balance, but we can look at them from another viewpoint—a perspective that takes us out of the body. When we look at the illness called cancer, we may be observing a condition that comes almost entirely from troubles that have not been handled in a manner that is constructive. We may be seeing the destructive side of response to stress in one's life.

Workers in cancer support groups have known for years that the more loving and caring that such a group provides—whether they are family, friends, or an established group—the cancer patient lives out his or her life, instead of gradually dying through the remaining days.

A recent medical study showed how a large group of cancer patients responded with or without a support group. David Spiegel of Stanford University reported to the annual meeting of the American Psychiatric Association how a group of women with breast cancer who received group therapy and lessons in self-hypnosis lived an average of almost twice as long as a similar group who were given only traditional medical treatment. The study involved eighty-six women who had metastatic spread of the cancer. The support group women lived an average of 36.6 months compared to 18.9 months for those not taking part in a support group.

In the Edgar Cayce readings, in the Christian Bible, and in practically all of the world's major religions, survival and healing are closely related to the divine plan and to the love that is tendered to those in need. If the ministrations and caring and the love and tenderness manifested in a support group do not fully heal the patient from the illness—as has happened in the scriptures and in daily life in this and other countries—then the least such caring is likely to do is to make the individual more comfortable, more hopeful with the knowledge that someone truly loves him or her, all of which brings about an extension of life.

Love is a powerful aid in the healing process.

When one goes through the process which we call healing, perhaps the mind is experiencing rejuvenation as the body is healed. It could also be a scar on the soul that is undergoing the process which we designate as healing—a process we can call an adventure in consciousness.

Whether it's one or the other, an awakening to the soul's direction and destiny is almost always involved. Cayce had much to say about healing. The following extract is a good example and may give us insight indeed as to why support groups are valuable:

> For it is true that the body mentally, the body physically, should be and is capable of resuscitating and revitalizing itself, if it is raised in spiritual direction for the activities of disturbing conditions in the body.
>
> Hence mind over matter is not to be lightly spoken of, nor is there any disparaging remark to be made as to the body-physical being revivified, resuscitated, spiritualized such that there is not [any] reaction that may not be revivified. (1152-5)

Sow the seeds of kindness, helpfulness, long-suffering, gentleness, patience, brotherly love; and leave the *increase* to the Father, who *alone* can give same either in the spirit, the mind *or* the body.
Being patient even as He. (1472-3)

INCOORDINATION IN HEALTH AND DISEASE

Being patient may, in and of itself, prevent a person from experiencing a degree of incoordination in his or her body. To grasp this concept, we need to explore the ways in which someone's body may be incoordinated.

One year I went to Virginia Beach and decided to do some research on the topic of incoordination. I asked my son Bob, who was volunteering in the A.R.E. Library at that time, to research the index to the readings and give me a list of those readings where incoordination of the body was identified.

The list I got back was fifteen pages long with three columns of reading numbers on each page! I was discouraged about doing exhaustive research on the subject. I was not very patient, and I suppose part of me was at least a bit incoordinated as a result of my frustration.

I did discover, however, that there are many ways in which the body becomes incoordinated, and there is a significant relationship among stress, incoordination, and body malfunctions. I also found that Cayce, in his readings, identified this quality so consistently that we need to understand what we think of as a basic lack of balance in the functioning of the human body, or what Cayce calls "incoordination."

In the terminology of medical neurology, coordination is described as the combination of nervous impulses in motor centers to insure cooperation of the appropriate muscles in a reaction. The word itself comes from the Latin *cum*, meaning "together with" and *ordinare*, meaning "to regulate." In relation to the body and its function, this definition seems not only adequate, but almost poetic: "The harmonious activity and proper sequence of those parts that cooperate in the performance of any function."[36]

Cayce's readings would seem to agree both in essence and in fact with such a definition of coordination. The lack of coordination would mean illness in the human being, much as its presence means balance and health. In the following reading, one of the symptoms is nausea. This certainly is a reflection of the lack of harmonious activity of the stomach and the other related digestive organs, which usually function in harmony and cooperation to produce a feeling of ease and well-being rather than the tendency to regurgitate:

> Occasionally—once a week or oftener—the Jerusalem artichoke should be a part of the diet. This will tend to correct those inclinations for the incoordination between the activities of the pancreas as related to the kidneys and bladder. These as we find, even in this form, will make for better corrections . . .
>
> *(Q) What causes frequent periods of nausea and what can be done to overcome this condition?*
>
> (A) This, as we have indicated, arises from the incoordination between the upper and lower hepatic circulation, owing to the disturbance in the pancreas with the kidneys. For, as will be indicated and found by the body, when such occurs there is the more frequent activity of the kidneys *and* the bladder; and becomes rather as a nervous reaction.
>
> Hence the precautions in the directions as to diet, to change the activities of the circulatory forces in relation to these, will bring better conditions and a removal of the causes of these conditions. (1523-7)

Perhaps the greatest difficulty for the physician is to understand how we might work with the lack of coordination between the pancreas and the kidneys, for instance, or between the upper and the lower hepatic circulation. In the above reading and others, a concept of relationship emerges which states that there is a working together, a cooperation, among various parts of the body and various activities of those parts that seem on the surface to be completely unrelated. This concept presupposes not only a communication among those parts or activities, but also a consciousness in them that can be part of the communication.

In every activity of the body organs or systems, there is a higher control which calls for a working together under normal healthy circumstances. When one part becomes ill or disturbed, there is the beginning of bodily illness. In the reading quoted above, there is that higher direction that controls perfectly the relationship and coordination between the pancreas and the kidneys *when conditions are proper.* But when a lack of working together comes about, a further complication ensues—the imbalance or incoordination between the two parts of the hepatic circulation— and this produces the nausea.

Such a cause and effect is not thought of in the practice of medicine. This concept is one of the ways that the Cayce material, taking into consideration the reality of the spiritual nature of humanity, brings to mind another perspective when we view the reality of the human body and its activities.

Another fascinating concept represented here is how a simple therapy, such as a dietary change, can bring about normality in the relationships of the consciousness of the organs of the body. If we were discussing people who were in disagreement, we would think that there would need to be thoughts exchanged and agreements reached. Cayce looks at things from the perspective of this being a material world, and material changes that are reasonable can bring about a body/mind/spirit change and healing results.

The castor oil packs, however, are suggested as the beginning therapy for the condition described partially in the following reading:

> As we find, there are disturbing conditions as prevent the better physical functioning in the body. These as we find arise from specific disturbances that have upset the glandular system, as related to coordination between superficial and the deep circulation in the eliminating system. There is the involvement of the activity of the lymph and emunctory circulation—or what might be called lymphitis. (2643-1)

This woman had been diagnosed by her physicians as having Hodgkin's disease, a condition that Cayce describes as lymphitis. He saw in this woman an incoordination between the superficial and deep circulation of the eliminating system. Emunctory means excretory, so this particular problem is involved with the lymphatic circulation throughout the body, both in the deeper parts and in those near the surface. Keep in mind that the lymphatics are part of the immune system of the body, so the incoordination affects the proper function of a part of that activity that protects our bodies, rebuilds the body in a sense, and brings about the very first steps in elimination of body cellular wastes—which takes the wastes to the general circulation and then to the skin, lungs, kidneys, or liver and intestinal tract for final disposal.

In this instance, incoordination, lack of cooperation, and malfunction are all involved in how the body functions more properly.

As incoordination applies to the study of the castor oil packs, however, the most commonly discussed incoordination in the Cayce readings is between the autonomic and the cerebrospinal nervous systems. This, in turn, is related often to the lymphatics and to the circulation mentioned above.

Keep in mind the definition of coordination as being the harmonious activity and proper sequence of those parts that cooperate in the performance of any function, and let's look at some of the comments in the readings about lymph, nervous systems, assimilating system, and circulation.

Now as we found, there are disturbing conditions, and they arise from incoordination; as produced from the lack of that *within* the system during the period of pregnancy to carry the full flow of coordination between the lymph and the activity of the sympathetic and cerebrospinal system.

Hence in those areas about the assimilating system, without great precautions, we have that breaking of the connection between the active forces of [nerve] *impulse* and the *ability* to carry same out in physical reactions ...

As we find, with *consistency,* there may be help brought; but it will require patience *and* persistence in the application of those influences and forces as may bring a better activity in the vibratory forces of the nerve *impulses* of the body ...

First we would apply the heavy castor oil packs for at least three days, each time before the corrections are attempted. Apply these heavy castor oil packs an hour each day, over the liver and caecum area, all along the right side; that we may break up those tendencies that cause this incoordination there. (1790-1)

In case 1790-1, the disturbance in lack of coordination apparently comes between the lymph and the already coordinated two nervous systems, causing a weakening of nerve impulse in the whole body, not only to the muscles of conscious activity, but probably also to functions of organs, glands, and unconscious smooth-muscle action throughout the body.

Cayce probably saw the function of the packs as eliminating "tendencies" toward incoordination by stimulating better lymphatic drainage, liver function, and autonomic activity.

Coordination exists among the nervous systems and the activity of the blood in the body's circulatory system. Wherever a blood vessel makes its way through the body, not only in the thoracic and abdominal cavities, but also throughout the arms and legs and the somatic tissues of the trunk, it carries with it the nerve supply which constricts the vessel or makes it dilate. These are the sympathetic and the parasympathetic nerve supply, respectively, although it is known that some portions of the blood vessels receive their muscle dilators also through the sympathetic.[37] Interestingly, we find that the peripheral blood vessels, including those which supply the extremities and the somatic tissues of the trunk, are innervated through the sympathetic fibers derived from the sympathetic trunk ganglia. These fibers join the spinal nerves through their sympathetic roots and reach the blood vessels through branches which join them at intervals along their course.[38]

We thus see the necessity to the body of the autonomic supply and some of its function, and, by inference, the importance of the balance offered through the cerebrospinal nervous system in its relation to the autonomic. Cayce indicated that these two systems meet intimately in the spinal cord or the sympathetic trunk ganglia, and that is where a coordination with the blood supply is created.

This means that when an incoordination exists here, the blood vessels do not perform their varied duties well, thus bringing about certain disease conditions of the body. This is rather well illustrated in the following extract of a reading taken on a forty-four-year-old woman, whose case number is 5266.

> There have been those operative forces which have allowed, or caused, adhesions and lesions to form in areas where the cerebrospinal and sympathetic nervous system and blood supply coordinate, in the brachial areas especially.
>
> The results have been, and are incoordination and a form of anemia that will be hard to combat unless certain measures or precautions are taken.
>
> These conditions, as we find, might be termed accidents, in that there were, in the healing of the body, conditions where nerve tissue or tendons became involved, and thus the circulation especially in the upper extremities is such that these have become useless, in a manner, in comparison to their normal activities.
>
> This is by pressure, and through the adhesions and lesions formed there are those conditions producing the complications such that nerve and blood supply are not receiving their proper stimulation for the activity and circulation, from the adhesions.
>
> Glands are involved in this. Thus, we have a progressive activity of incoordination, of poor circulation. (5266-1)

So, as we saw earlier a lack of balance or coordination among the lymph and the nervous systems, we are shown here the same sort of bodily upset among the circulatory system and the nervous systems.

I think it is necessary to make it clear that Cayce understands the human body as having awareness even at a cellular level. Thus, systems are a collection of consciousnesses and act together much like a city acts as a unit.

Coordination in this light becomes more of an understandable activity. But at the same time it is seen to be even more necessary to be present and working.

In the cases I reviewed (see Part II) where castor oil packs were used, the most striking incoordinations Cayce found were between the autonomic and cerebrospinal nervous systems. A relationship must exist within the body between these two systems. We see it in action today in the emotion-related diseases, although most of the discussion at an academic level of physiology deals with the functioning of each system, rather than the way the two systems might work together in a coordinated effort.

Cayce indicated, however, that lack of proper coordination at this level was deeply involved in the causation of diseases as widely diverse in their apparent etiology as multiple sclerosis, appendicitis, anemia, hemiplegia, and grand mal epilepsy. It would seem worthwhile to look more closely at examples of these and attempt to reconstruct the underlying philosophical concepts which might be linking these disease entities together.

A forty-eight-year-old man, later diagnosed as having multiple sclerosis, was given a series of readings. Interestingly, it wasn't until the second reading that he was given the suggestion to use castor oil packs. However, some detail of a physiologic nature is to be found in the first reading, which is quoted in part:

> ... we are speaking of:
> *The blood supply,* this indicates that there was first an unbalancing in the metabolism of the system, and congestion through the activities of the assimilating forces or system as related to liver, pancreas, spleen, and a lack of coordination with the excretory forces of the liver.
> And for same, as we find, there have been misap-

plied conditions. Hence we have had an infection arising, producing . . . through the nervous system—a breaking of coordination between the sympathetic or vegetative and cerebrospinal nerve systems.

This accounts for the irritations to portions of the superficial circulation, as well as the inability for the body to rest, also for the impressions the body receives of disturbing influences and forces about the body.

It is not a mental condition wholly, yet its reaction to the sympathetic system, through the sensory reactions, gives that very reaction to the *bodily* functioning in the system.

Hence the arthritic reaction at times, the conditions as effects to the sensory organisms—both the auditory as well as to the vision; for all become a part of the general disturbance. (1623-1)

Here we see an incoordination between the assimilating system and the excretory system, at least that part represented by the liver. This apparently caused a toxic condition which precipitated the incoordination between the autonomic and the cerebrospinal nervous systems.

Cayce indicated that the autonomic ganglia, which are found alongside the spinal cord but outside the spinal canal, are "centers" where most of the coordination between the two nervous systems is localized. In case 1623, these were unduly sensitive at times.

Apparently, to follow the inferences in the reading, this break in coordination must be found in the upper ganglia which supply sympathetics to the visual and auditory apparatus, as well as farther down anatomically, where the organs of the body receive their nerve supply. Here also is seen in one person a rather amazing group of symptom complexes, which Cayce states all come about as the direct result of what he calls a break in the coordination between the autonomic and the cerebrospinal nervous systems: superficial circulatory disturbances, insomnia, probable psychoneuroses, arthritis, and auditory disturbances.

Here are conditions which nearly everyone has had to one degree or another. Also there are symptoms which have nothing to do with the motor system of nerves—the nervous system which has to do with locomotion and conscious activity. Yet, according to these readings, the result of poorly coordinated systems of nerves represent, in one sense, the means by which the conscious mind acts in the body on the one hand and the system through which the unconscious mind acts on the other. This idea has much support, not only in the Cayce readings, but in the already explored physiology of the body.

ATTITUDES, EMOTIONS, AND INCOORDINATION

The field of psychosomatic medicine, pertaining to the relationship between the mind and the body, has led into what today is called psychoneuroimmunology. This, in turn, has shaped our present thinking more into the belief and understanding that emotions, attitudes, and feelings are closely associated with disease processes, not only resultant from them but in many cases causative.

Perhaps we will gradually accept the fact that emotions cause physical changes through glandular outpourings of hormones from several of the internal secreting glands and increased flow of energies, especially over the sympathetic nervous system. With such an acceptance, we will more completely see the oneness of the body with the mind and we will begin to associate our physical bodies more with the mind and the spirit within.

Presently, however, this is still a difficult concept to accept. We are not ready to look at an appendicitis, a kidney infection, or a thyroid disease and admit that attitudes of mind in relation to our friends or our family, an emotional flare-up with a father or a sister could possibly have anything to do with causing this physical disease, in spite of the fact that we do accept a stomach ulcer as a sign of emotional or attitudinal imbalance, as well as many other conditions.

Cayce found that emotions were, in at least some cases, the primary cause of the incoordination between the autonomic and the cerebrospinal nervous systems that we have been discussing. The following instance, case 5240, is an example.

This fifty-one-year-old woman, if her letters are to be understood correctly at a psychological level, was very critical in her nature and she continued to be so even seven years after her reading was taken. Such an attitude is perhaps one of the most difficult to overcome and, at the same time, causes perhaps more trouble to the body through creating stresses and an easily upset nervous system. Cayce suggested a simple regimen to overcome the asthenia which the woman was experiencing, but he apparently also was aware of the woman's resistance to changing her attitudes, the cause of the whole thing, so his most important recommendation was almost in an aside:

Also, there has been, and exists in the present, incoordination between the nerve systems of the body. An overanxiety, a fear has caused overtension in the nervous system, especially as related to the areas in the upper dorsal or through the brachial centers, and has caused a great shock to the body, so that the ability of the nerves to coordinate in replenishing energies through the circulation has caused this great weakness which exists in the body.

These may be materially aided but it will require as

much activity of the mental self as those administrations from any mechanical or medicinal natures. (5240-1)

Background on this individual was supplied in a letter seven years after the reading was given. She stated that the shock which Cayce described was an "emotional upset, partly caused by a half-crazed principal with whom I was unfortunately working after my thyroidectomy when I was weak. In his mental weakness (he had suffered severe mental trouble and I had of necessity filled his office), he had the idea I wanted his position and was more than unjust and cruel."

She had a thyroidectomy six years before the reading. She also had experienced chronic appendicitis attacks, which were relieved, according to her letters, by castor oil packs suggested in the latter part of her reading. She followed only partially the suggestions made for the relief of her tiredness.

This case adds somewhat to our understanding of what Cayce called incoordination of the nervous systems. It is one in which we do not find a severe disturbance of the locomotor system as in epilepsy, but rather an underlying condition to be found within the body organs. It is almost as if Cayce were saying that when these systems become incoordinate, the energies may spill outward into the conscious cerebrospinal system, causing an uncontrolled overflow of energy as in Parkinsonism, for instance. These same energies may deviate inward and spill over, so to speak, into the unconscious-autonomic area of nervous activity, creating dysfunctions of various types, such as in the case we have just discussed. These can be minor or very severe, partially or not at all controlled.

The importance of this incoordination in the cause of illness, as seen by the sleeping Cayce, cannot be overemphasized. He repeatedly involves it in his own peculiar type of physiological discussions in explaining how the sicknesses come about. He repeatedly sees the sympathetic trunk ganglia as being the major area of coordination between the autonomic and the cerebrospinal nervous systems. And he explains, time after time, the widespread ramifications of this incoordination as they are manifested throughout the body.

We can examine these rather minutely if we look again at reading 2643, given for a thirty-four-year-old woman who had Hodgkin's disease. This case is also interesting because the woman who requested the reading followed the suggestions completely and was free from all symptoms and signs of the disease.

Four years later, however, she had a relapse when she resumed quarreling with her husband. The marital situation disintegrated, the Hodgkin's recurred, and the woman, depressed, refused to return to the use of castor oil packs and other suggestions which initially helped her. She passed away from the illness. Following is a partial extract of this case, which is quite complex and lengthy, but which adds much to the present subject under discussion:

> There are areas in the spinal system where pressures on those centers of coordination between the cerebrospinal and sympathetic nerves leave the ganglia so relaxed as to at times fill the superficial areas with the fluids that should be circulated through the system by the very impulse of activity of the circulating system itself. Thus the variation in pressure. Hence the heart, liver and kidneys become involved. These vary as to their activity under varied pressures . . .
>
> As there has gradually grown to be a variation as to the areas affected through the cycle of activity of the organs, by pressures in various portions of the body, we find that the impulse of this fluid reacts either to

the feet, knees, hips, abdomen, lung, extremities—
arms, face and neck—any of these, or all of these may
be involved at once, with some particular area out-
standing, as there is the pressure being carried along
the reflex impulse in the areas of the colon and the activity in the coccyx end of the spine, as well as that
indicated in the 6th and 7th dorsal in the body.

That (the 6th and 7th dorsal) was the first area involved, from an injury some four years ago—a wrench
or a pressure produced in that area; combined with an
injury to the end of the spine.

These have been, and are, as we find, the sources of
the disturbance. That there has not been greater involvement to the functioning of the organs of the body
is an indication of rather the nature or character of the
sources of the disturbances to this glandular force as
related to the supply of lymph produced in the body.

Thus there is indicated a cold area over portions of
the abdomen, through the glandular activity of the
lymph ducts and glands through digestion. While
there is apparently little association of the activity of
the nervous system in digestion and the lymph activity in assimilation, we find that these are the
sources—and pockets of lymph through the intestines. Thus those times when there is such soreness
through portions of the abdomen and the jejunum, as
well as the colon itself, in those areas of the caecum,
the ascending and transverse area of the colon. All of
these at times give disturbance or distress, either at,
before or following those changes that are wrought by
this accumulation of lymph in any of the areas of the
body. (2643-1)

Etiology, the original source of disease, becomes sometimes unique in these readings, as we see above. Apparently

the injury to the spine, at the 6th and 7th dorsal areas, combined with that to the coccyx (the end of the spine), was the basic cause of this process which is called Hodgkin's disease.

In addition there are pressures thus produced on what Cayce calls the centers of coordination between the cerebrospinal and the sympathetic nerves. Anatomically, this would seem to mean either the anterior or posterior roots of the spinal nerve, including probably the dorsal root ganglion or the spinal ganglion, as it is often called, or the white and gray rami communicantes, as they leave the spinal nerve and join the sympathetic ganglia. These latter are the connecting links between the sympathetic and the spinal cord, but anatomically would seem to lie out of the way of pressures which might come about from vertebrae which might be malaligned with each other, a condition which is termed subluxation: incomplete dislocation.

To follow the thoughts above, it would seem logical to understand Cayce as stating that the pressures thus evolved caused the sympathetic ganglia to be "relaxed"; that impulses for proper function and tone of the arterial, venous, and lymphatic systems were not present. The incoordination, then, might be understood to derive from pressure on the anterior and posterior spinal nerves and the dorsal root ganglia, these being the centers of coordination referred to.

This whole concept, stated here in such an incomplete and undoubtedly obscure manner, is not found anywhere in the textbooks of neurology, anatomy, or physiology as they exist today in the field of allopathic medicine. The theories of osteopathy and chiropractic are not within the scope of this discussion, although it can be said that both schools of healing have as a primary thesis that subluxation of vertebrae, one upon the other, is causative of disease, and correction of such malalignment will aid in or bring about directly the cure of the abnormal body process. To further

clarify the situation, it can be said that Cayce was un-
schooled in healing. In his recommendations, he used all
types of therapies, apparently without discrimination as to
source but with considerable discrimination as to result.

Returning to the patient with Hodgkin's disease, we see
the disturbed function of the autonomic system reflected
in the circulation, the heart, liver, and kidneys and the fluid
imbalance (probably through the lymphatic system) having its effect in the face and neck, the arms, lungs, abdomen,
hips, knees, and feet. Also, we see mentioned the resultant
lack of coordination between the autonomic nervous system in its digestive capacity and the lymphatic system in its
role in assimilation of foodstuffs. The distresses and
sorenesses coming about through an accumulation of
lymph in pockets throughout the intestines is part of the
picture that Cayce sees within the body of this particular
person afflicted with what we call Hodgkin's disease.

It is not difficult to begin to comprehend that Cayce's
understanding of the body and its diseases had much to do
with relationships and with the functioning of the system
of nerves that we call autonomic—the system that works
according to the make-up of our unconscious minds: our
fears, greeds, desires, hates, jealousies, contentions and our
hopes, beliefs, loves, and faiths.

Chapter Eleven
A Professor of Anatomy and an Unconscious Mind

WE ALL LIKE A CHALLENGE, ESPECIALLY IF it is in an area of endeavor with which we are very familiar. Cayce was given such a challenge in June, 1943, when he was asked for a reading by a medical school professor of anatomy who became case number 3056. This physician was sixty-eight years old at the time, and he had suffered a paralysis which caused him to give up his teaching. His attending physician's statement was as follows:

May 20, 1943

To Whom It May Concern:

This is to state that I have attended Dr. [3056] for the past year.
He has had mitral insufficiency on a rheumatic basis

*since youth. For the past ten years or so he has had au-
ricular fibrillation for which he has taken digitalis
with good results. Occasionally a mild degree of
anasarca sets in, easily controllable with increased
digitalis and salyrgan.*

*Four years ago he suffered a sudden left hemiplegia,
probably on an embolic basis, which has persisted.*

*Recently he has had neuralgia involving the right
shoulder and arm.*

*Blood pressure 130/80, pulse around 80, totally irregu-
lar. Loud systolic murmur over apex, lungs clear, no
edema at present.*

> *Sincerely,
> (signed)
> John Cannon, M.D.*

Here was a man whose life was spent in institutional
medical instruction at a high level, with knowledge of the
human body far superior to most people at the time. Would
the reading which Cayce was to give change in its nature
and become more orthodox in its language, would it use
more conventional terms, and would it deviate from its pre-
occupation with coordination, nervous systems,
assimilations, and the like? This was indeed a challenge.

I have included most of the information given which
lends itself to diagnosis as Cayce would understand it. The
therapy includes castor oil packs, but there are numerous
other suggestions which are not pertinent here. This is a
monologue between an unconscious mind and a professor
of anatomy.

As we find, there are disturbances that prevent the
body from its better physical functioning. These have

to do primarily, we find, with that coordination between the sympathetic (or vegetative) nerve system and the cerebrospinal nerve system.

Thus the bursa are involved that are in those areas dealing with locomotion, or controlling of the locomotory centers, almost crosswise of the body.

While the effects produced are much like those from a leakage, hemorrhage, or the like, we find that these have *not* been caused by what is commonly called a stroke. While many of the organs are primarily involved, we find that the greater part of the distress arises from other sources than that ordinarily involved in such conditions.

These, then, are conditions as we find them with this body, [3056] we are speaking of, present in this room:

While the activities in the blood supply, the elements as related to the hormones of the blood force itself, indicate disturbances in activity, and the slowing of circulation through portions of the extremities of the body, these are *not* the effects as of the body of the circulation itself being involved.

As we find, then, more of the involvement is in the nervous systems, the energies of the body, the activities of the body having been such as to break down that proper coordination between the nervous systems; that is, the cerebrospinal *and* the sympathetic (or vegetative) systems, as indicated.

Because there have been those disturbances that weakened the centers or ganglia along spinal areas, where the activities between the superficial and deeper circulation were involved, the effects produced are in the locomotories that were and are controlled by the energies that are controlling from the central nervous system, the central blood supply, and the superficial blood supply.

Thus we find these conditions existing through this body:

The brain forces and their reflexes are active. These are near normal, save as they are disturbed by pressures that exist in the areas of the 5th and 6th dorsal, as through the sympathetic control, the activities in the locomotion to the left upper portion of the body. And there we have an inflammatory condition that causes pressures which prevent nerve impulse that flows with the blood supply through that portion of the arm, as to cause the lack of the activity of coordinating usage of same.

We have in the 2nd lumbar that which prevents coordination of that flow to the right side in the lower extremities. These are not so inflamed, but are of the nature that causes the lack of the reflexes in the use of the nerve and muscular forces of this limb.

By the activities of the body that brought about these conditions, there has been the lack of that assimilated from that digested, through the activity of glands, to supply sufficient of the elements for producing the stamina—or the impulse in the nerve body itself, the impulse for the retraction, or reaction, or reflex from the brain; the gray and the white matter in nerve itself.

As indicated, these do not extend to the spinal cord nor into those areas that would direct the impulses to activity of the organs—either the kidneys or the liver. While both come into reflex reaction, and at times become involved, these are not cut off. Neither is there caused that which would bring about atrophy; indicating then that this involvement is more to the sympathetic connections with the cerebrospinal system, at centers or ganglia indicated in the body.

The lack of this element, with the overuse of the energies of the body, both as to locomotion in the lower and upper portion, causes these areas to suffer under this stress and strain.

To be sure, there are involvements—from the long period of inactivity—to the heart, the lungs, the liver and the kidneys. But these as yet are secondary to the disturbance in the superficial, the lymph and the emunctory circulation, that is involved through the activity of the sympathetic nerve reflexes; which control not only secondarily the organic activity but that as related to the imagination, the sensory reaction, and the impressions that go to make up those reflexes in the responses to impulses from activity of the sensory centers.

These, as we find, may be materially aided—if those elements are added to the system that are the basic effect of activity of nerve, muscle *and* impulses that go to supply sufficient activity in the vibrations of the body force itself.

For, all activity is of an electrical nature. (3056-1)

Cayce indeed gave an anatomical-physiological monologue worthy of a professor of anatomy. He met the challenge by using the same method of approach we have seen him already use. His diagnoses seem to be a lack of proper assimilation of elements needed for nervous tissue regeneration, incoordination between the cerebrospinal and vegetative nervous systems, improper function and "weakening" of the sympathetic ganglia, and a vague glandular imbalance which affected the assimilation of foodstuffs. One might add to this a neuritis, if the inflammation he mentions can be assumed to involve sympathetic connections to the spinal nerves.

Apparently Cayce saw these conditions as being the underlying causes of what the professor's attending physician called mitral insufficiency and auricular fibrillation from rheumatic fever, anasarca (severe edema or swelling of dependent portions of the body due to accumulation of fluid in the intercellular spaces—lymph), left hemiplegia (or paralysis), and a neuralgia of the right shoulder and arm.

It is certainly difficult to draw conclusions from this reading which would carry any note of finality. However, certain comments are worthy of consideration at this point.

Let's try to analyze it in a language that is more comprehensible to the professional and to the lay mind. There seems to be a continuity of concepts which have already been discussed and which persist in designing a physiology of the human body that has all the earmarks of being different in philosophy and function from what is presently considered valid. Yet it is only in subtle ways that there appears a divergence of ideas.

To review Cayce's "diagnosis" of this man's illness, we find that there is first mentioned that incoordination between the cerebrospinal and the vegetative nervous systems. This is the primary disturbance. Then Cayce describes an inflammation of the sympathetic ganglia which correspond to the 5th and 6th dorsal spinal nerves. His description leads one to believe that the inflammation perhaps involves not only the ganglia, but the rami communicantes—these on the left side of the spine in the thoracic cage. He indicates that this inflammatory process prevents the normal flow of impulses through the vegetative nerve supply to the blood vessels and that which goes with the blood vessels to the entire left arm.

Starling has shown that all the vasoconstrictor fibers of the body have their connection with the cerebrospinal nervous system through the ventral roots of the spinal nerves from the first dorsal to the third or fourth lumbar inclusive.[39] These centrally derived nerves connect with the sympathetic system in the ganglia of the sympathetic trunk. He has shown likewise that in dogs, the central vasoconstrictor nerves to the forelimbs leave the spinal cord and enter the ganglia by the fourth to the tenth thoracic nerves.

There are fibers which also cause dilation of the vessels, these being parasympathetic and sympathetic in origin. Thus, in many parts of the body, the sympathetic nerve supply produces both actions usually attributed to the sympathetic on the one hand and the parasympathetic on the other.

Cayce implies that the inflammation in the 5th and 6th dorsal sympathetic area brings about a lack of sympathetic nerve impulse through this just-described vasomotor system to the left arm, and that this lack produces in some strange way an inability to coordinate the use of the arm musculature. This type of end result is not described to my knowledge in the medical textbooks, although it can be seen from what has been discussed in the past few paragraphs that the sympathetic disturbance which Cayce describes could have a basis in anatomic and physiologic fact. What is not understood is that such a disturbance could bring about any sort of incoordination between the autonomic and the cerebrospinal nervous systems, or that it could bring about an inability to coordinate the muscles of an arm into coherent activity.

Related to the above is Cayce's next diagnosis, which points out a similar difficulty—although not strictly the same—in the right leg. Trouble in the 2nd lumbar sympathetic ganglion causes difficulty in the use of the right leg as it deals with the nervous control and the muscular activity. There is no inflammation here, however.

Cayce's next comment relative to the professor's physical ailments points out that there has been faulty assimilation of the foodstuffs due to improper endocrine function. This deficiency brings a weakness of the impulse in the nerve pathways between the brain and the body areas. This doesn't occur in the spinal cord, but in the autonomic nervous system, which again brings us back to the sympathetic ganglia and the rami communicantes. This is the anatomical location of what we might call "the sympathetic connections with the cerebrospinal system." He points out that since this is not in the spinal system itself, there will not be atrophy in the tissues; that the liver and the kidneys will not be involved because the sympathetic supply to these organs is not cut off or severely disturbed. Rather, he points out, they are only occasionally involved in the patient's symptoms and bodily dysfunction.

Cayce's insight of the professor's body next indicates that there is involvement of the heart, the liver, lungs, and kidneys of a strictly functional nature, secondary to inactivity and not really of importance yet. Rather, he points out that the disturbance in the ganglia with their associated (disturbed) sympathetic nerve reflexes have produced (1) a faulty superficial circulation to the muscles of locomotion in the trunk and extremities; (2) a lymphatic circulation that is not functioning properly; and (3) an upset "emunctory circulation," or blood supply to the organs of elimination, perhaps—for this reference is unclear.

However, the more important point in this particular paragraph is that, although the sympathetic supply of nerve impulses and reflexes controls the activity of the organs themselves and is thus quite important, the real, primary control which is exercised here is that over the function related to the imagination of the mind itself and the "sensory reaction" and related to the impressions of the mind which formulate the reflexes brought about from sensory receptors (afferent sensory impulses). An example of this would be the drawing away suddenly when a finger touches a hot object.

Obviously, there are statements and references here that dangle, like an undesirable participle, when one begins to put together the statements in this reading into a semi-understandable form. Yet in this reading there are a whole group of challenging ideas which seem to continue to relate the whole body and its mental faculties, conscious and subconscious, into a coherent unity.

We cannot leave discussion of this case without pointing out the rather obvious fact that Cayce did not mention the mitral insufficiency and fibrillation which had apparently resulted from rheumatic fever at some earlier time. Nor can we easily understand his discussion of the abnormal function of the right leg since the attending physician's statement didn't make reference to it. However, Cayce's other references are consistent with the medical diagnoses submitted, if we allow for different modes of approach to understanding what has occurred within a human body that has not been explored surgically.

Chapter Twelve
Our Bodily Functions "Uncontrolled"

The Autonomic Nervous System

CASTOR OIL PACKS HAVE TAKEN ME IN MY therapeutic efforts with my patients all the way from the misery of a sprained ankle through the agonies of an inflamed perineum to the discomfort of a stiff neck. At this point we need to understand the nervous system at more depth. In doing so we will see a parallel between the anatomy and physiology of medical science and that found in the Cayce readings.

Initially visualize the nervous system as a whole as having its central and dominant control located in the brain, but with other subcortical areas of control elsewhere in the body. Nerves arise from all of these areas in a vast network penetrating all parts of the body and having control over movement and function in a tremendously complicated outflow of energy or impulse which is called efferent. This network brings back—to the various ganglia, to other centers of the body, and to the brain—similar energy impulses which, when received, produce awareness, what we call consciousness, in the human organism. This is termed afferent nervous activity.

While nothing in the entire nervous system is really simple in its construction or in its activity, I shall try to simplify this discussion, realizing that such a procedure opens the door for error in statement and in communication.

Since it is my object to primarily discuss the autonomic functions of the nervous system, I won't dwell long on the central nervous system. We know that the cerebral cortex is the seat of all higher activities of the mind of our thought or of our consciousness processes. The frontal areas of the brain particularly are related to these associative functions. Consciousness, as we know it, seems to be brought into being physiologically through or accompanying the passing over of impulses from the afferent to the efferent side of the cerebral arc.

Starling[40] describes in terms almost poetic the mind function in the cortex as it deals with consciousness, sense, and memory:

"The states of consciousness glide continually from moment to moment in an unbroken stream of experience, consisting of a sharper focal content with a fringe of slighter definition and leaving behind it a trace which we know as memory. By a process of attention we can single out parts of the stream of consciousness for closer focusing.

"There seems but little doubt that our conscious experiences are the result of complex integrations of sensory impressions, which are assessed by being checked and compared with traces of previous experiences."

We are also aware that the brain directs all our conscious

physical activities and that it has an influence over—although not directing—those parts of the body that work under an autonomy of their own, the so-called vegetative functions of the body.

The nervous system may be divided into different parts and has been in the past. Anatomically, it might be divided into the central nervous system, consisting of the brain and the spinal cord, and the peripheral nervous system, including the cranial and spinal nerves with their respective ganglia and the peripheral portions of the autonomic nervous system.[41]

While the above definition with its divisions might prove helpful anatomically, the functional or physiological understanding of the nervous system is better arrived at through the use of a functional classification. Such classification gives us a clear distinction between the autonomic nervous system, which controls the so-called vegetative functions that are beyond or beneath the level of the conscious mind,[42] and the cerebrospinal nervous system, which includes the brain, spinal cord, and all the efferent nerves that are associated with consciousness and control-conscious activity.

This leaves a large portion of the nervous system to be accounted for the afferent flow, without which there can be no cerebral arc, no phenomenon we call consciousness. This might be called the sensory nervous system, since its function subserves all five senses.

These afferent impulses do not all reach the cerebral cortex. Some are intercepted at a lower center or ganglion where a type of integration or association occurs, producing again a function through the efferent system. In this manner the functions of the organs and tissues of the body are controlled.

This efferent division, which we call the autonomic (it controls the functions of all tissues except the contractile states of the striated skeletal muscles through the ganglia distributed throughout the body), has been called by many names.[43]

Because he believed it to control the sympathies of the body, Winslow in 1732 introduced the term *sympathetic*. Bichat came along in 1800 to call it vegetative, to designate its control over essentially nutritive as opposed to "animalic" life processes. Gaskell in 1916 introduced the adjective involuntary, contrasting its activity with the voluntary system governing the body musculature.

Langley in 1921 suggested the phrase which we now use widely—autonomic nervous system—to designate the entire craniospinal innervation of visceral as well as somatic vegetative functions, to stress the fact that outlying ganglia, while dominated by the central nervous system, nevertheless maintain a measure of independence or autonomy. This system was subdivided into two portions: (1) the sympathetic in a restricted sense, including the fibers arising from the eighth cervical to the third or fifth lumbar segments of the cord and ganglia; and (2) the parasympathetic embracing (a) the tectobulbar fibers leaving the brain stem with the third, seventh, ninth, and tenth cranial nerves and (b) the fibers emerging from the second to fourth sacral regions of the cord.

These two systems have in common the possession of synaptic connections situated in pools called ganglia which lie outside the central nervous system. The important bodily functions which are mediated through this system of nerves and ganglia are of much greater physiological significance than its modest anatomical build would lead us to expect.[44]

Thus we see a tentative framework of the nervous system as a whole, divided for functional purposes and for reference in this study, into (1) a cerebrospinal, (2) an autonomic or vegetative, and (3) a sensory nervous system. This arbitrary division, while perhaps not completely without errors of omission, gives us a starting place from which to evaluate those functions in the body with which we are concerned in dealing with sickness and health and to look at the relationship between these systems as they pertain to organic function, its breakdown, and its restoration.

When relating our minds to our bodies, we first observe that we think we are in control of everything we do: we get up out of bed in the morning when we want to, alarm clock or no alarm clock, we comb our hair, we eat food, we use the telephone, we drive a car, we do our daily work, we are businesslike or friendly. All these things we do by choice and can do them consciously, when we want to. And, of course, all this is so.

However, closer observation shows us that there is something quite unique about these bodies we have and that we think we control. There are portions of our bodies that are *uncontrolled*, that function without our thinking about them or how they work. And these functions—such as digestion, heartbeat, kidney, liver, or pancreatic activity, to mention a few—may act up in such a manner at times that the *controlled* body is incapacitated by that which we call *uncontrolled.*

It is this latter situation which I will explore further: the uncontrolled body or, more accurately, the nervous system which mediates this "lack of control" which the conscious mind recognizes. This nervous system, of course, is the autonomic. We shall try to understand better its activity in the body and primarily how it relates to the other two systems: the cerebrospinal and the sensory.

The term *uncontrolled*, of course, is inaccurate when applied to the bodily functions that are ruled by the autonomic nervous system. It is important that we realize that these functions, in reality, are controlled within ourselves. They are not under the direction of the conscious mind. Thus, by definition, they must be under the rule of the unconscious mind. The emotions of the body interfere with autonomic function to a minor degree at times and in a drastic manner at other times. Thus, again by definition, our emotions must be classified with the unconscious mind. Our conscious thinking mind with its choice, on the other hand, rarely interferes with bodily function. Only occasionally is conscious thought of such a nature and direction that it breaks down the barrier between the conscious and unconscious and stirs the emotions.

Yet, emotional interference with various functions of the body implies that there is another direction of an integrative nature that regulates life activities within the body and maintains—we hope—a state of health most of the time.

This direction, this control, this mind can be located anatomically in the various nerve plexuses and ganglia which make up a portion of the autonomic nervous system, just as the brain is considered to be the anatomical location of the conscious regulating mind of the "controlled" activities of the body. This mind is called, in our present understanding of the body, the unconscious mind. It contains not only the emotions, desires, drives, and instincts which are considered to be basic to human nature, but also the inherited tendencies which we see as racial and familial characteristics.

In addition, the unconscious mind contains the ideals and high purposes which seem to be inherent in those individuals who have striven to great heights of accomplishment and service to their fellow human beings. All these attributes—and undoubtedly more—are part of our unconscious mind and represent that which, in reality, rules the portion of the body functionings which we have just termed the "uncontrolled."

This act of grouping body, mind, emotion, and aspiration gives a more comprehensive picture of what might be going on within our bodies at an unconscious autonomic level and gives us a comprehensive picture of this particular nervous system as we investigate it and try to understand it.

Reede, in 1918, published a fascinating discussion of the autonomic nervous system as it relates to dermatology.[45] Here is his opening statement:

"The archetype of the vegetative or autonomic nervous system is found in the ganglionated or metameric nervous systems of the lower vertebrates, in which in the absence of a forebrain and prior to the development of intelligence or consciousness the necessary functions of life are carried out through a few simple ganglions and nerve fibers. In [humans] this primitive nervous system has been long disregarded because lost sight of in the study of the evolutionarily superimposed forebrain or cortex, with its highly organized association systems and central nervous system extensions. The activity of the vegetative nervous system still takes place below the level of consciousness and independent of intelligence, but it nonetheless sways the very foundations of life."

We can see from the above quotation how we, in our evolutionary relationship to the lower vertebrates, have developed the forebrain which becomes the means by which consciousness or choice or whatever factor that allows us to be dominant over all the other animals of the earth can be experienced. It also reminds us that many of the functions of life, learning, aspiration, and direction which we find in ourselves can be demonstrated without the higher consciousness symbolized by the forebrain. Remember that lower vertebrates lived, functioned, caught their prey, and escaped from enemies without the higher integrative centers.

The endocrine glands are directly involved with autonomic function as they are also deeply related to emotional expression. In performing its function to regulate and coordinate metabolic activities in the body, the autonomic nervous system acts not only through direct nervous impulses of its own, but also through its association with the endocrines. These ductless glands have a certain degree of autonomy, but the larger part of their activity is in direct response to the call of the vegetative nerves.[46]

Not only does a ductless gland respond to the stimulus of the nerve, but its secretion, in turn, reacts on the nerve, making it still more sensitive in function. In this connection, it is interesting to note that the medulla of the adrenal gland, which is the gland of "fight or flight" of the sympathetic division of the autonomic nervous system, morphologically corresponds to a sympathetic ganglion.[47] The medullary hormone is known as adrenaline. This substance is also found mediating the discharge of sympathetic nerves, along with a closely allied substance, norepinephrine (demethylated epinephrine), in varying proportions throughout the body.[48]

Much could be written about the relationship of the sympathetic and the parasympathetic nervous systems. To summarize it or condense it leaves many questions unanswered, in addition to those which physiological research has not yet solved. Present-day physiology and pharmacology perhaps see these two portions of the autonomic nervous system as basically antagonistic functional units but working together all the time, while we are awake or asleep, to keep a physiological balance in the body.

The sympathetic nervous system equips the body, in its full action and through the phenomenon known as irradiation, for the intense muscular action required in offense or defense. It is a mechanism of war which mobilizes all of the existing reserves of the body.[49] It accelerates or heightens function and prepares one for emergencies or emotional crises of any sort and becomes, in this way, an exploiter of energy. However, it is not always intensely active; rather, most of the time it is controlled in its function, creating a constructive force throughout the body in a balance with its counterpart, the parasympathetic.

During hours of sleep the sympathetic activity is at a low ebb. This can be ascertained by looking at the absence, while asleep, of the results physiologically which can be observed in the body when the sympathetic mobilizes for action. In sympathetic stimulation, the eyes dilate and the rate and force of the heart are increased. The muscles, heart, lungs, and brain receive a markedly increased flow of blood as the blood pressure is increased; but the blood vessels are constricted and the blood supply to the other internal organs of the body is markedly decreased; the hair stands on end and sweat pours from the sweat glands of the skin; body temperature usually increases. The sphincters are contracted and the intestinal peristalsis is inhibited.

These changes in the body are obviously absent when a person is resting, at peace with the environment, or asleep. This condition points up the rather interesting functions of the parasympathetic nervous system. When the sympathetic is relatively dormant, then its counterpart, the parasympathetic has to be relatively dormant. Thus we find the heart rate slowed, the body temperature decreased, the blood pressure lowered, the pupil constricted, the blood supply shifted from the muscles, heart, lung, and brains to the organs of digestion, assimilation, and excretion, and the motor activity to these structures increased. This allows for proper elimination of wastes, proper utilization of the saliva and digestive juices and the activities of digestion, and the further proper absorption or assimilation of digested material into the bloodstream and lymphatics of the body.

All these activities come about through the functioning

of both the cranial and the sacral portions of the parasympathetic. The sacral gives innervation to the large intestine from the splenic flexure distally and to the generative organs, the sphincters, and the lower urinary tract. Generally speaking, the cranial division supplies nerve energy to the remainder of the functioning organs. Thus we can see why it has been said that the cranial division of the parasympathetic nervous system performs the tremendous service of building up body reserves and fortifying the body against times of stress and need, while the sacral division supplements the cranial by cleansing the body through ridding it of its urinary and intestinal wastes.[50]

Because of the intricate functional make-up of the two parts of the autonomic nervous system, we tend to group them as separate entities, so to speak. We should hesitate, however, to do this simply because the source of the neurons is different and the function is apparently antagonistic.

We note, for instance, that they are not really so antagonistic as one would think on first consideration. Rather they augment each other by their reciprocity[51]—like two hands holding a basketball. We also see that there are areas of the body which receive both adrenergic and cholinergic (as parasympathetic stimulation is called) supply through the medium of the sympathetic nerves.[52]

Functionally, we see a difference in the nature of the two systems, but it is well known that an individual animal in the laboratory can live and procreate with all of the sympathetic nervous system plus the adrenal gland removed.[53] That there is higher cortical influence to this entire system, of course, must be recognized in evaluating the autonomic. We are probably safe in assuming that much still remains to be learned about the functioning of the nervous system, particularly this portion.

All pre-ganglionic nerve fibers of both parts of the autonomic nervous system arise in the spinal cord or in the brain stem. The sympathetic pre-ganglionic fibers synapse with ganglion cells in either one of the sympathetic trunk ganglia or ganglia located in close proximity to abdominal or pelvic viscera. The parasympathetic pre-ganglionic fibers, however, proceed until they near their final destination—often in the wall of the organ or structure—before they synapse with a ganglion cell.

Other fibers, known as post-ganglionic fibers, proceed from the ganglion cells. These are more numerous, at a ratio of 32-1, than the pre-ganglionics.[54] The interesting fact is that acetylcholine is the chemical substance which mediates all of the pre-ganglionic connections of the autonomic nervous system, as well as being the substance that is released at the post-ganglionic nerve ending. Acetylcholine is found in all the sympathetic ganglia and in the medulla of the suprarenal gland.

The significance of this seems obscure at first glance, but there are some relationships here to concepts which appear in the Cayce readings that this volume addresses. Cayce has treated the autonomic system as a unit, not acknowledging any division in functions. He also has spoken of those connections to the cerebrospinal nervous system. We see from the preceding material that the cerebrospinal nervous system is connected to the autonomic through the pre-ganglionic nerves in both sympathetic and parasympathetic. Assuming that these pre-ganglionic fibers actually belong to the autonomic nervous system, we would see a relationship between the cerebrospinal and autonomic nervous systems being affected with one type of nerve only, which releases acetylcholine at its nerve ending and which acts as the mediator, then, between the conscious and unconscious minds at a physical level. The autonomic afferent nerves, of course, are those which are part and parcel of the sensory nervous system and are distributed not only to the ganglia but also to the spinal cord and then to the brain.

Cayce repeatedly discusses electricity as the motivating force in the human body, and he sees this transport of information in the nervous system as an electrical phenomenon mediated by a chemical. Such a view indicates that all these synapses are really controlled by the thought or the activity of the electrical impulse wherever instigated by the consciousness of the person. This approach requires another look at how these impulses act in the daily activities of the human being and, with such an examination, provides us a solid foundation for understanding the use of castor oil packs.

Chapter Thirteen
Under the Impulse of These Ganglia

STRESS PLAYS A PROMINENT ROLE IN TODAY'S SOCIETY. All of us feel its effects in everyday life, and individuals in positions of responsibility sometimes suffer extremely from the effects of stress on the human frame. Laboratories have been designed to search into the mechanisms of stress and to find ways to prevent it or alleviate its effects. The Christian church offers as its antidote to stress the application in one's life of a simple concept called faith. Cayce, in his readings, made infrequent use of the word *stress*, but he commented constantly on its activity in people's lives as he described their physical bodies and what was going on inside them.

In the course of his internal description, Cayce referred to the autonomic nervous system in nearly every instance as it related to other functions within the body. In the reading he gave for a forty-three-year-old man who was exceedingly tense, Cayce described functions of organs as being under the direction or impulse of ganglia, especially those found in the sympathetic trunk alongside the spinal cord:

> IN THE NERVOUS SYSTEM, that the body from the mental portion has been under strain is evidenced by the characterization in many of the centers along the cerebrospinal nervous system, especially in those ganglia along the 3rd, 4th and 5th dorsal centers. WITH the unbalanced condition in the elements of the system, the organs that function *under the impulse of those ganglia* [author's emphasis] or centers show that there is a congestion at times in the FUNCTIONING of digestion and assimilation. This within itself shows, or indicates, how that the disorders in this physical body become, then, as complications that COULD arise, were there not the equal balance brought in the mental, the physical, the imaginative body. (4393-1)

Cayce indicates through several other readings that these centers or ganglia play a much more important part in the functioning of the body and especially the autonomic nervous system than just directing the organs and their workings. In his unconscious state, Cayce indicates that these ganglia are, in fact, the brain where mental processes take place, where sometimes the physical (as well as the physiological) activities of the body itself can be controlled through mental ability. He poses an idea which is far-reaching in its implications: that the sensory system, as he calls it and as we have understood it, has a closer association and more potent effect on the autonomic nervous system than it does on the cerebrospinal.

This means that all of the sensations which come into our bodies, no matter from what source, primarily affect our unconscious minds, our autonomic nervous systems, and subsequently the whole of the physical body that is supplied by the autonomic. These portions of our being are more sensitively affected than our conscious mind and our physically activated body. We then become more complicated because these afferent impulses which we call sensory include voices that we hear, stories that we read, television shows that we watch, odors that we smell, and even food that we taste. In addition, we need to add the variety of impulses that arise from the ways in which we are touched physically and the various organ and internal sensations that arise from either an internal disturbance or a sense of well-being.

Is it any wonder, then, that a hypnotic voice or a simple odor, for instance, can bring about changes in secretions of the stomach, just as in Pavlov's dogs? Or is it strange that a summer breeze caressing one's skin brings an uplift in spirits inside, or the odor of a perfume causes an excitement of a nature difficult to describe? These are part of the workings of this body we live with daily. Cayce described these activities in their abnormal workings, which were the causes of the bodily illnesses in the individuals who came to him.

A man, in treatment in a mental hospital for schizophrenia, was given a series of readings. In the fifth reading Cayce's source gave a lengthy dissertation that described what was going on within the man's body. The reading tells a rather comprehensive story, touching not only on the bodily conditions, but also on the effects of the special type of low electrical vibration which had been described earlier for his use.

That there may be understood just what is taking place in the mental and the physical reactions, and their coordinations in the system, it would be well to review these reactions; that those who care for the body, and those about the body, may know that with which they have to deal—and that to be met!

As we have given, there is a very good mental reaction—as far as the mental being is concerned. There is very good reaction in the physical body. The trouble is in the *coordination* of these through the various centers. Nerve exhaustion, through conditions that were of the nature as we have described, prevents the coordinating much in the same way and manner as where an electrical connection is made with a system and is only partially, or spasmodically, *made*—as it were—to make connection; by mental reaction or mental suggestions, or by physical reactions. Then, they are only partially connected, so that the reactions are very much in the same way and manner.

Now, in the physical forces of the body (as seen and understood, in the nervous systems of the body), there are those glands that secrete fluids which in the circulation sustain and maintain the reaction fluid in the nerve channels themselves.

There is the cerebrospinal system, which in this body is *very* good.

There is the sympathetic nervous system, which makes for the *impulses* and the reactions that are received in the system by suggestive forces, by reactions that make for stimuli to nerve centers and plexus through the system that make for connecting with the cerebrospinal to the brain centers themselves. For, all impulses for reaction must have their centers, or reacting centers, in the brain centers themselves.

Now, in the cerebrospinal system there are centers, or ganglia, where there are those connections with the cerebrospinal that go more directly to the brain. And we find that all [of the] sensory system are more sympathetic with the activities of the sympathetic, or the sensory and sympathetic system—see?

Hence by speech, by vision, by odor, by feeling, *all* make a sensitive reaction on a body where there is being electrical stimulation to ganglia to make for connections in their various activities over the system.

Hence it may be easily seen how *careful* all should be, how much precaution, patience and persistence must be had, in making every suggestion; by speech, by sight, by feeling, by vision, by eating, by sleeping, by *all senses* of the body; to coordinate with the *proper* balance being made in the system. See?

Hence, with the low form of electrical vibration that is set up in the system, there is being sent out from these ganglia those infinitesimal *feelers*, as it were, that will gradually make connections with those ganglia and centers in the system that have been destroyed by the reactions in the system which destroyed gland functioning for the creating of these fluids, by those activities that have been seen. (271-5)

In the following reading which was given for case number 3990, the first for this individual, Cayce elaborates a bit on how he sees this sensory system relating to the autonomic:

The cause lies here to the sense of hearing and to the eye. The sensation to the system, on the sensory system, on to the nervous portion of the body is through the sympathetic system. The nervousness in the system or in any body, produced by the sensory system, of course, is stronger, and more tiring to the whole physical body than that of a nervous force produced from the cerebrospinal system, because that acts on the organism of the make of the man. That is, through the sympathetic or abnormal mind, and through the mind of the body in itself. (3990-1)

In the following reading, the tables are turned, and the sensory system is affected by the improper functioning of the sympathetic:

The functioning of the sensory system we find very good, save the strain as is put on the system when the sympathetic nerve system becomes overtaxed from the condition in the pelvis. The effect is more noticeable to throat and eyes, for the higher vibration of nerve force from sympathetic is affected by the overtaxing. (3712-1)

The causes of disease, of course, are multitudinous, and we are all well aware of this.

We often blame such causes on bacteria, viruses, weather changes, air conditioning, and our heredity, to mention a few; but we avoid like the plague (which we respect) attributing any causation to our emotions. We may be willing to accept the idea that anger, for instance, could cause disturbance and perhaps disease in someone else, but in me? The conscious quirks and make-up of all human beings permits us to overlook it in ourselves, while seeing it full-fledged in our neighbor. The presence of anger, yes, we see and admit, but causing trouble? That's another question. Cayce sees in the following reading a group of conditions that were brought into being when "during such time there was much anger in the body (this she understands better than others.)" (42-1) It apparently precipitated conditions wherein there was sensory-sympathetic communication at times when this should not happen. Perhaps this might explain some of the symptoms patients bring to their physicians, symptoms which are usually explained away as being imagined or psychosomatic. This reading is a bit difficult to follow, but informative:

In the nerve system, in this we find the greater
trouble, physically, in the sympathetic nerve system,
for the refractory nerve centers in the system show
how this system is magnified in its action in the body;
that is, in those centers where organs function through
the physical action, and become the involuntary action, such as digestion, sight, pulsation, heart's action,
the body unconsciously has reached the condition
where it must, with its voluntary forces, keep all functioning. That is, occasionally, and often, at times keep
on its mind that all *must* function rather than being
the condition of a normal body, functioning normal,
for the organs are organs nominally . . . Then the force
of the sympathetic act, as it were, to control of the
body. It is through such reaction from sympathetic system that the sensory organism often gathers the
reaction through the abnormal functioning of all of the
sensory system; that is, often the body sees, feels, hears,
recognizes conditions not perceptible to the ordinary
functioning of the normal sensory system . . .

The organs of sensory system abnormal in the conditions as given, through the action of sensory and
sympathetic nerve system, coordinating when they
should not. (42-1)

The sensory system, as we see it formulated in the readings, assumes prime importance in the daily living process.
Certainly it is more important for those who are seriously ill
than it is for healthy persons to be certain that sensory impulses of *all* natures are soothing, rather than disturbing, as
they are channeled into the consciousness of the individual
concerned: sounds of nature rather than sounds of the city;
pleasing and uplifting colors rather than those that are dull
or discordant; music that inspires or makes happy rather
than music of warlike or emotional concept; absence of

sharp sounds or traumatic emotional happenings; applications to the skin which would bring a resting and receptive state; food that is prepared well and is simple, not exotic, and appeals to the taste normally rather than being of a gourmet nature; odors that speak of Thanksgiving rather than of the nearby bar.

These perhaps are a few of the choices that must be made in relationship to sensory input surrounding a sick person. The spoken word, of course, assumes primary importance, since it is through this mechanism that humanity achieves its greatest degree of communication between one individual (or center of consciousness) and another. The human being, you will remember, is the only one on this planet who can carry on a verbal relationship with another at a creative level, using words in all manner of ways. This is our prime difference from other beings. Thus words as received through the senses are critically important for they convey ideas, concepts, motivations, and so often emotional content to the hearer.

It is not surprising to see instructions like the following, then, for a schizophrenic:

All suggestions about the body should be of a *constructive* nature; the love influence that comes from within every heart, mind and soul, that would build for *creative* forces without selfish motives in same. (271-5)

Among the extracts from the readings which should be quoted are those which give us bits and pieces of understanding of the true physiological concept of the nervous system as it exists here, for study reveals that there is a consistency and continuity of thought and idea throughout the readings related just to this question. The following two extracts point up some of the characteristics of the sympathetic system with its ganglia as they pertain to their role of governing functions or being as a brain. The readings also indicate a more vague reference to the cerebrospinal, which is not easily understood at this point.

As indicated, this deterioration is not in the cerebrospinal system, else we would have mental deficiency, but is in the secondary brain, as it is ordinarily called, or the brain—as it were—of mental processes. Then, those centers along the cerebrospinal system that are called the sympathetic or vegetative nerve forces have been, and are, deficient . . . of those elements or vitamins . . . needed . . . (294-212)

. . . we find that these have at various times suffered under various ways and manners. Sometimes these have taken on the form of a disturbance between the cerebrospinal and the sympathetic system in such measures until the body would almost break out in a cold sweat, but from what—the entity could not determine within itself. At others it became cold and clammy and shaky in various portions of the system.

This is a reaction to not only the sympathetic or vegetative nerve system (which is the double system that runs along the cerebrospinal and functions for the coordinating or the governing between the mental body and the physical body), but to the cerebrospinal system (which is rather the deeper nerve forces that supply energies to the various portions of the body, the organs and the locomotory centers, for responses).

Hence he passed through a period when as much disturbance to the body was the inability to recall or remember or to know just what the reactions or things were that were going on about the body; forgetting, as it were, very easily, and at other times when he wanted to forget he couldn't. These were not mental aberrations; they were the effect of the two nerve systems, as it were, warring one with another owing to the poisons that have been allowed to accumulate . . . (1055-1)

Mental illnesses, such as psychoses, give us a good opportunity to study the relationship between cerebrospinal and the sympathetic or vegetative nervous system, if indeed these are the areas where the conscious and the unconscious minds reside. The psychotic individual shows a splitting of personality, a drawing away from what we call reality, and a complete lack of what psychiatry calls "insight." This is an inability to comprehend what is wrong or, more dramatically, that there is anything wrong with himself or herself. In true psychosis, there should be a relatively complete break in the communication between the sympathetic and the cerebrospinal nervous systems, if what has been discussed thus far has validity. A case in point is helpful:

One girl, a thirty-two-year-old artist, was apparently sexually attacked by a man who invited her to his apartment on the ruse that he wanted to buy some of her paintings. She may have been given very strong suggestions afterward by the same man to repress the entire incident, which was an exceedingly traumatic affair. She broke down and was institutionalized with a diagnosis reported by her family to be insanity. A more accurate diagnosis would probably be an acute depressive psychosis.

There being in this body, with this entity, a high nervous temperament, with ideals as high, as keen as may be found in many a day, the activities through which the entity passed have shattered its hopes, its aspirations—by the advances that were unspeakable to the entity, the *mental* self, the higher self.

And in the attempt to escape, and finding self

trapped as it were, the physical exercise and activity in the attempt shattered the connection between the cerebrospinal and sympathetic system; especially in the coccyx and the lumbar areas.

Losing consciousness the entity became a prey to those suggestive forces as were acted upon, and by the injection of outside forces to keep that hidden as attempted upon the body.

Then, in its present environs, there have been only moments of rationality; and then *no* one to respond brought greater and still greater depression to the better self...

The impulse of the imaginative system must be quieted through gentleness and kindness, yet positiveness. (1789-1)

This gradually becomes an understandable concept—the idea of this suddenly induced psychotic state being a shattering of a physical and electrical connection as well as of a mental state of being. The etiology—trauma of a physical and psychogenic nature—brought into the coccygolumbar area a physical condition that might be described as a breaking apart of nerve connections. This is certainly a fascinating manner of looking at this type of illness.

I've found that Cayce does not see this as an unusual cause. The following case seems to be quite similar in nature. This man had been treated in an institution and was apparently either ready to be released or was just released when the reading was given. Prior to his illness he had a post office job, but apparently his family had been advised that he had been turned down for re-employment because of his mental condition (called in the correspondence a nervous breakdown). Since his partial recovery, however, he had not been advised by his family that he would not be re-employed.

Yes, we have the body, [1513].

Now, while we find there is a better coordination between the mental and physical reactions in this body, unless there are other applications to keep this coordination, or to supply the activities to the nerve energies of the system, we find that with the realization that there is an improbability of being restored to active service [in his job] the condition would become very much disturbed again.

For through pressures upon nerve energies in the coccyx area and the ileum plexus, as well as that pressure upon the lumbar axis, there has been a deflection of coordination between the sympathetic and the cerebrospinal nervous system. (1513-1)

This shows a "deflection" rather than a "shattering," as in the prior case. Apparently this person was not as ill as the female artist. But it is interesting and probably significant that in both individuals there came about a coccygolumbar area injury to the connections between these two nervous systems. Apparently, as the readings pose the information, this area is a common one for localization of etiology for mental derangement.

That the coccyx is involved actively was not left in any way questionable in this reading, and the question-and-answer portion which follows shows us some of the fineness of adjustment which must come within the body at times to bring about a state of balance and health again.

(Q) Is this coccyx misplacement the direct cause of the condition?

(A) As indicated, this was the direct cause of the condition—as combined with the general deflection produced in the system by same, see?

Hence the necessity, with the correcting of same,

that there be the vibratory forces to re-enliven, or to enliven nerve ends where coordination comes *between* the sympathetic and the cerebrospinal systems.

Hence the necessity of the inspection occasionally, as indicated. (1513-2)

Let's look, however, at what might come about from a normal balance of the autonomic nervous system, rather than the more disturbed examples of a lack of coordination.

We know some of these from other fields of study. For instance, the study of dreams in recent years has shown that there is a marked increase in the physiological activity of the body concomitant with the activity of the unconscious mind in dreaming. Heart attacks, peptic ulcer reactivations, asthma—all these diseases which are known to be related to emotion and stress—occur more often during the dream state. Likewise, the autonomic functions are different in these different conditions. For instance, there is a great upsurge of activity in the sensory system coming from the organs of the body during the dream state which does not exist during other sleep states.

We are undoubtedly justified in also observing that those individuals who experience what we call visions are seemingly in an altered state of consciousness when this occurs. Although, to my knowledge, there has not been a reported study on whether these individuals have an altered physiological state during these periods, I would be inclined to believe that they would have such an altered state, based on what I have researched from the readings.

The conscious mind and the will of an individual, through self-suggestion, self-hypnosis, and positive thinking certainly get into the unconscious in ways that control bodily functions. This happens with many who are not even aware of it. Cayce describes this sort of thing in the two readings that follow:

With, by, and through the *mental* ability of the entity, or body, to *control* self, the sympathetic system has often controlled the physical forces of the body, for the body often finds self in this position: If it would allow itself it could fly all to pieces in a moment, but keeps itself much under control of the mental forces, through the sympathetic system—yet at times this reaches the point where almost nerve exhaustion exists. Hence—rest—quiet—these have often been that factor in the recuperating forces of the body, yet has never corrected that as produces the condition. (943-1)

In the blood supply, we find this in very good condition, considering the effect the assimilation has on the system and the functioning organs, for the will and mental forces of the body gauge the effect that this has through the sympathetic nerve system to a great extent, and diverts much of the condition that might be created in the system.

. . . In the connection between the sympathetic and cerebrospinal nerve system, we find the sympathetic above that of the ordinary, or above normal. Hence, we find this body discreet . . . in its manifestations of conditions that affect the body in any manner, and through this controls the body much to the betterment of conditions . . .

Might be many things said. The body is exceptional in the functioning of sympathetic, that especial center of the soul and mental forces. (4359-1)

Cayce indicates here that the sympathetic nervous system is the center of the soul and what he calls the mental forces. Earlier we learned that he described it as the center of mental processes. He certainly ascribes to these structures of the body a specific, dynamic, and dramatically important function which is probably more clearly shown in the next two selections from the readings:

> The whole system becomes below the normal action of all its functioning powers, yet no organ itself becomes particularly involved save in the slowing of the action of the whole system, everything becoming, as it were, drugged into its dormant condition of becoming to the separation of the action of cerebrospinal forces as is the seat of the physical and the action of the sympathetic forces which is the seat of all of the soul and spirit forces. See? (4595-l)

> In the mental forces of the body, we find as in these. The activity of the mental or soul force of the body may control entirely the whole physical through the action of the balance in the sympathetic system, for the sym-pathetic nerve system is to the soul and spirit forces as the cerebrospinal is to the physical forces of an entity . . . (5717-3)

What is the soul and spirit force or forces? Perhaps a definition is not to be found in the realm of neurology. However, we can sense a better understanding of how the soul and the spirit may be operative within the body when we begin to put these bits of psychic readings together into a comprehensible whole (as each reader should do for herself or himself) and see the wide vistas of understanding that begin to grow within. Where within? Perhaps as an impulse passes an associative center, crosses over from the conscious-cerebrospinal by means of a pre-ganglionic fiber, and rests in some cells of the third or fourth ganglion of the sympathetic trunk.

Chapter Fourteen
What About This Oil That Heals?

FOR PURPOSES OF SUMMATION, LET'S SUP-
POSE WE LEAVE open and undecided the basic
assumptions which the Cayce readings explore about healing and the nature and function of the body, especially as it
pertains to the use of castor oil on the body.

With such an open mind, we can look at these concepts
of healing with a certain amount of candor—granting that
they could be right or wrong, but evaluating them in light of
information derived from various sources.

All these concepts, of course, would relate to the manner
in which castor oil affects the human body and how healing
of that body takes place.

Some questions concerning these ideas would be:

1. What is this energy that we call Life or Life Force?
2. Where does it originate?
3. What is the intelligence that lets cells and organs function according to their "nature"?

4. What relationship is there between our endocrine glands and our emotional responses?
5. How do our emotions directly affect the organs and systems of the human body? What about "healthy" or "unhealthy" emotions and their effects?
6. What is the nature of "unconscious" direction of the vegetative functions of the body?
7. What part does the autonomic nervous system play in this?
8. Do we really create illness or health in our own bodies?
9. What then *is* healing of the body?

So, what about this "oil that heals"? Is it really the oil that does the trick? Could it be the hands that lovingly apply the pack or the oil to the body? Medical treatments using drugs often simply force an issue—it kills the bacteria or moves a physiological or biochemical activity toward what is desired by the doctor. Rarely does it bring healing by itself. Does castor oil bring such healing or is there a subtler activity going on?

IS HEALING A MOVEMENT
OF THE LIFE FORCE?

Cayce suggests that all healing of any nature is a new awareness in the consciousness of the cell or organ which leads toward a oneness with the Creative Forces of the Universe; an awakening, an arising above the nature of the earth into the nature of that which created the earth. Cayce often said that healing of any nature is to bring to the consciousness of those forces within the body an awareness of the Creative Forces or God. The story of seventy-two-year-old Velma, recounted in Chapter Five, may be an example of this healing process, as discussed in answers to the following questions:

1. What is this energy that we call Life or Life Force?
2. Where does it originate?

3. What is the intelligence that lets cells and organs function according to their "nature"?

As you may remember, Velma came to the Clinic in 1988, having had a hysterectomy twenty-three years earlier. Since the surgery, she had constant gaseous distention, constipation, abdominal "miseries," edema of the ankles, and episodes where her "gut" would feel as if it were twisting in on itself.

She returned to the Clinic two weeks following her first visit, after starting on castor oil packs, and gave us this report: Within minutes after the very first pack was placed on her abdomen, she felt as though the gut untwisted on itself. From that time forward, there has been absolutely no return of the symptoms she had earlier experienced—no twisting sensations in her gut, no ankle edema, no abdominal miseries, constipation, or gaseous distention. All were gone after twenty-three years!

The nature of life as it is seen in the readings is fascinating and can be traced in the Bible. God created you and me in His image. God, we know, is Spirit, and thus we also are spirit in our original form. As souls, He created us with minds, gave us life through that life force we call spirit, and along with that gift, He blessed us with that great power—and His greatest gift—which we call will, the power to choose.

The spirit is that life force, the energy, which gives us the power to do whatever it is we choose to do, using the power of choice. So, within us, in the temple of our own bodies, can be found a power greater than the universe itself, for it is there that God has promised to meet us.

That power, originating as the manifestation of God, gives us inherent intelligence in all parts of our bodies—the consciousness of knowing how to perform functions which those individual cells or organs are designed to do and thus keep us totally healthy.

We have consciousness and awareness throughout our

bodies, and it is always consciousness that we are dealing with when we talk about or deal with the healing process. Cayce frequently said that there is consciousness even in the atom.

If God created leaves in the trees, the brooks that bring us water to drink, and the atoms that make up the oxygen we breathe, then there has to be that knowledge within our bodies, within those atoms themselves, which help to make us even more wonderful than we think we are.

Perhaps the seventy-two-year-old Velma accepted the healing nature of the castor oil and made the quantum leap within her own consciousness from being tied to the earth consciousness to being in attunement with her real self, the soul body, in this particular experience.

Our bodies, then, *can* function according to the intelligence and awareness that is their true "nature"—the manner in which our soul bodies were created in the first place.

If we follow our true "nature," then we are tuning in to the manner in which we were originally formed, in the image of God. Our experiences on the earth, however, have led us to stray from that origin and align ourselves more closely with the earth plane, which we have not yet been able to overcome. This may be how illnesses are brought into reality. It may also be that when we do overcome the earth, we will be in line to return to our origin, which is always our destiny.

WHAT ABOUT OUR GLANDS, OUR EMOTIONS?

It is well known that the endocrine glands have a direct effect on the physical body through the autonomic nervous system and through the hormones that are released through the bloodstream. Let us consider, then, the following:

4. What relationship is there between our endocrine glands and our emotional responses?

5. How do our emotions directly affect the organs and systems of the human body? What about "healthy" or "unhealthy" emotions and their effects?

It's not difficult to understand how these relationships occur. When an impulse is sent out from the adrenal gland, for instance, the message affects every functioning cell in the human body. Likewise, the hormones that follow the initial fight/flight response from the adrenals are poured into the bloodstream and fortify, in a sense, the message which the nerves have already broadcast; that is: "Get ready for a fight!" All the glands are alike in that they have both nerve and hormonal activity.

Each of the glands has a particular nature that we call emotional. The sex glands, for instance, are well known, though little understood regarding their emotional content and effect on the body. It is well known that emotions grounded in one of the sets of glands can be constructive or destructive in their nature.

The Cayce readings had much to say about that. One such statement bespeaks of the absence of courage and faith:

> Fear is that element in the character and in the experience of individuals which brings about more of trouble than any other influence in the experience of an entity. For, when ye are sure of the right path and follow it, ye do not fear. (2560-1)

The positive side of this glandular function is courage and faith—where fear does not exist. It is interesting to follow the sureness of the right path, suggested in the above reading, in the instance of Richard Disney.

Richard had read my book[55] and "had to write this letter" to me. The reason had to do with his following the path he was sure of, even though it looked at times as if it was not right. He had faith! This is his letter:

"I have a history of back problems stemming from a football injury I received in 1964. I had surgery in 1965 and again in 1980 to remove parts of a crushed disc.

"In November of 1987 I hurt my back again, and went to a chiropractor for an adjustment. I was out of work for several days, showed improvement, and returned to work. I started suffering sciatic pain a few weeks later which radiated down my left leg. For the next month, I visited the chiropractor four more times, had bed rest, electrical stimulation, Motrin®, aspirin, Tylenol®, ice, heat, massage, etc. Nothing seemed to help. Actually the pain got worse.

"I am a member of A.R.E. and my wife and I both enjoy reading Edgar Cayce material. My wife, Ellen, was reading your book about the castor oil packs the same day I had given up and gone to a regular doctor. The doctor set up an appointment for me with a neurosurgeon for the next day. The evening before I went to the surgeon, Ellen applied a castor oil pack for one hour to my lower back.

"I felt some relief, but was still in a lot of pain. At this point, I was convinced that surgery was the only course of action left. The surgeon examined me, set up a myelogram, blood work, and x-rays for the next week. My wife continued applying castor oil packs with heat.

"After seven days of castor oil packs and a few doses of olive oil, however, the pain was completely gone. So, I cancelled all appointments. After a two-day break, Ellen once again applied the castor oil packs, this time for three nights.

"I have not had any reoccurrence of back pain or sciatic pain. We also used the castor oil pack on a cyst that my wife had on her leg. It started to drain after three applications and has caused her no more problems.

"I am convinced that I have experienced a miracle and I am thankful to my higher power, my wife's persistence and faith, and the information provided in your book at *just the right time.*"

There are always very important little details that are often missed when working with any experience or individual. In Richard's case, it involved the human being, his direction, his faith and love for his wife and her suggestions, and his belief that indeed Edgar Cayce did know what he was talking about, even though at one point it did not seem like it.

Nevertheless, Richard continued with the packs. There was not a hint of fear. The final result was like a miracle for him, although it was not, of course, a real miracle. It was part of the reality of energy and vibrations moving in such a way where there were no blocks in consciousness, and the result was healing.

THE UNCONSCIOUS MIND CONTROLLING THE AUTONOMIC NERVOUS SYSTEM

The memories of past lives, the residuals of the present-life experiences, all are to be found in the unconscious mind, somewhere in the reaches of the autonomic nervous system. The conscious mind, however, that brings about muscular movement and waking activity in this dimension has only vestigial relationships with the endocrine glands, the organs, and systems that keep the body alive. These latter are the domain of the autonomic and work under the direction of centers which have an autonomy—or a rule—of their own. This is the area where life is maintained and memories are kept for retrieval when needed. So let's examine:

6. What is the nature of "unconscious" direction of the vegetative functions of the body?

7. What part does the autonomic nervous system play in this?

8. Do we really create illness or health in our own bodies?

Edgar Cayce talked about the "vegetative"—or basic—functions of the body as being under the unconscious direction of the mind. These are the body faculties which keep on working no matter whether we are awake or asleep, are organized so that we do not need our conscious mind to tell them what to do. It is indeed fortunate that this is the case, for it would be impossible for our conscious thinking mind to tell the heart to beat seventy-five times every minute.

I think the direction was given to the centers of control in the autonomic probably during our intrauterine life, installed in a manner that we call genetic or under the direction of our genes and chromosomes. Very difficult to understand as to the method of installation, but very important to recognize as existing.

We can really think of the body as having three nervous systems, in order to simplify the manner in which the mind works.

The conscious mind, which allows me to write these words and makes it possible for you to read them; or which takes control of your going to work and moving your body around in whatever kind of activity you have chosen—this conscious mind works through the cerebrospinal nervous system. In the readings these nerves have at times been called the locomotor nerves.

The unconscious mind, on the other hand, has its activity through the autonomic nervous system in association with all the glands, all the organs, and all the other systems of the body. It indeed is given the responsibility of keeping the body alive and well.

However, the unconscious mind, as I mentioned earlier, is in touch with all memories, past lives and present, wherever those memories are stored. If there are patterns of emotion or attitude or belief that are out of accord with what we have chosen as our ideal, then there are problems in relationship among different parts of the life-giving organs. The controlling forces, one might say, have been confused. This can cause disturbance and will sooner or later bring about illness unless corrected.

The ability to know we are in this dimension is made possible through the five senses, originating for the most part from the cranial nerves. These are the nerves which allow our bodies to be aware of our environment and might well be called the sensory nervous system, although they are not recognized as such in physiology texts.

If there is created harmony in the reaches of the autonomic nervous system, then balance will come about in the physiology of the body, and health—rather than discord—will be the outcome. It becomes evident, then, that our efforts need to be directed toward that unconscious expanse of information that lies within us. For it is there that the secret of healing can be understood.

WHAT IS HEALING, THEN?

Healing, as it refers to the use of castor oil packs, has its alliance not only with the nature and functions of the body, but also needs to be understood in light of the fact that castor oil is composed of atoms, gives off vibrations, and has a specific activity on the tissues where it is placed.

In my own experience, I have found that castor oil placed over any part of the human being—or animal, for that matter—will stimulate the lymphatics to work more normally and will bring about a degree of healing through the stimulation of the immune system. Cayce suggested that use of the packs can and will affect the Peyer's patches and have a direct effect on the autonomic nervous system. A patient once told me that the pack was more relaxing than any tranquilizer she had ever used.

We now come to our final question to be considered:
9. What then is healing of the body?

At this time, we do not have enough information or research data to identify what healing really is or exactly how the castor oil pack brings healing to the body. However, I have found that simple treatments which interested individuals perform often give more good information about the method of activity and the possibilities inherent within their use than even the most sophisticated researches.

One such event involved a baby squirrel. Dolly Wijas gave me this story: "A couple of years ago we were fortunate enough to become the foster parents of a newborn baby squirrel. He was so small his eyes didn't open until after we had him home for two weeks.

"I faithfully fed him with an eyedropper and canned puppy milk every two hours. We also had a ferret, and that's where the trouble started. Being the 'natural' enemy of the squirrel, she got into his box one day and almost killed him.

"He had puncture wounds everywhere. We thought he was dead because he was totally limp and cold to the touch. Our vet, also a friend, said there was no hope. However, I had great faith in Edgar Cayce and decided it couldn't hurt to try castor oil wraps.

"I used an old piece of flannel, soaked it in castor oil, wrapped his body in it, and covered it with a heating pad. After twenty-four hours, his body was warm again and he would take a few drops of milk. Within three days, he was well on his way to recovery, and my friend, the vet, could not believe it.

"We kept him for about six months before he finally left on his own. It was a wonderful experience for our whole family—he taught us all a little more about love for nature and God's creatures."

This was healing from the castor oil and undoubtedly also from Dolly, who loved God's little creature enough to care for him. Is love a vibration? Castor oil certainly is. The oil also penetrates through the tissues where it is placed, so perhaps it brings about healing through the contact of a cleansing activity.

Another simple use, yet healing in its nature, came to me from another of our friends. She had broken her jaw in a car accident and her jaw had to be wired shut. She couldn't get rid of food particles that stuck to parts of the braces. She became concerned about cavities and gum erosion. She told me, "I was new in the A.R.E. and had read about all the benefits of castor oil. I decided to try brushing my teeth with a drop or two of castor oil on my tooth brush.

"The effect was all I could have hoped for. My teeth felt clean and the soreness from the wires disappeared. The end result was no cavities and minimal gum erosion."

There are literally thousands of stories I have heard about how castor oil brings healing to the body.[56] We may never know the whole story, but we must remember that this "oil that heals" was created by that Power which brought the entire universe into being and it was intended to be used to bring harmony and balance into the lives of individuals—both human and animal. For He loves all these creatures which He also created.

It seems to me that turmoil in one's life situation which needs desperately to be cleaned up may often result in turmoil in one's body where a cleansing should be going on, perhaps in the lower bowel or in one of the other organs that deals with elimination. I think we experience things more with symbolic portions of our bodies than we do with our so-called conscious minds. The real consciousness or awareness that we become involved with is most likely located in a specific area of the body. So cleansing of our lives might start with cleansing of the body, and this might be the *only* creative thing we can do.

Those individuals who are set in their ways will not often

respond well to the packs. Why? To those who will allow it, the oil brings peace to the body and to the consciousness. This is a measure of grace. Those who are set in their ways cannot let go of their own wills long enough to sense that it is the will of God that they be healed through grace.

Those who are receptive in their basic nature will benefit most from the castor oil packs. Why? Because being receptive is being as the little child. The child has faith without knowing why and so accepts all things as being the will and graciousness of God acting in his or her life. Peace comes to the child, throughout the whole of the earth—his or her earth!

Impatience destroys good results in this therapy for it unleashes the destructive activity of the energies of the adrenergic-sympathetic nervous system, overpowering the healing effect of the parasympathetic, as we know it.

Early conditions respond to this mode of therapy best, because the disturbed emotional patterns have not yet become solidified in the flesh. They have just left their fingerprints. Illnesses which require body change of a major degree—such as a fibroid or an ulcer or colitis of longstanding—to complete a recovery process requires patience and perseverance. The body has been seriously affected by those elements of consciousness which, for a long time, have acted detrimentally as a "normal" factor in the life pattern. These elements are not easily recognized and when found, are not easily moved out of one's pattern of awareness.

Healing may really be peace—a peace that comes to rest in the body, that is a reflection of the "peace that passeth understanding." We see it come to the body much as peace is allowed to come to the earth: a nation here and a nation there. When we find real peace in the earth, we may see a state of health having come to all bodies.

Part II

Case Studies

Introduction to Part II

I HAVE FOCUSED THUS FAR IN THIS VOLUME on castor oil packs and their use on the human body. We can see their use extending backward in time even toward ancient Egypt, where castor oil was used therapeutically. I have related these packs primarily with the field of healing, medicine, and parapsychology.

In studying their use as suggested by Edgar Cayce, we have discovered a man who could lie down and voluntarily enter a state of mind and body wherein his conscious mind was apparently not involved with what he was saying.

Cayce indicated that his entire autonomic nervous system was vitally active during this state and that the unconscious mind was that portion which was seeking out and reporting the information found. Often this information came from the unconscious mind of the other person involved—Cayce's client or patient. This condition directs us to the thought that we know already what is wrong with our bodies. We just can't reach down into that unconscious mind (or is it the autonomic nervous system?) and obtain the knowledge that we would like to have.

In bringing together all portions of my study, the inferences in the Cayce readings cannot be ignored. These inferences suggest that castor oil packs seemingly have a relationship with the nervous system, as well as with most of the other systems of the body, in their role of aiding the body back to health.

This brings us to the inquiry I made some time ago of their use in the general practice of medicine and my analysis, considering the value that may proceed from this study of eighty-one individuals whose varying conditions of illness were treated through the use of these packs.

These eighty-one cases are a random selection and represent only a fraction of the instances where we have used castor oil packs as the only therapy or as a coordinate therapy for one condition or another of illness. Some of the cases that have most impressed me with the therapeutic efficacy of this tool are not included. A continuing effort is being made, however, to collect more data.

My object in reviewing these cases in conjunction with the other information that has been presented is fivefold. It is certainly not a conventional research project. Many factors which are necessary for good, scientific research are not to be found here for a variety of reasons. What is to be found here, however, is information which is significant and case histories which are relevant to the purposes and objectives underlying this presentation.

My objectives are as follows:

1. To stimulate interest in this therapeutic regimen;

2. To show the exceptionally wide latitude of use that is possible with the castor oil packs;

3. To present and coordinate evidence that there is actual beneficial response in the human body to the application of these packs;

4. To discuss theoretical considerations relative to the action of the packs on the body; and

5. To begin to explore the validity of a unique understanding of physiological functioning of the human body, which is found in the Edgar Cayce readings.

CASTOR OIL PACKS IN APPLICATION TODAY

Much information can be derived from tables and statistics. However, a study of statistics too often removes us from the realm of human endeavor, even if, as Jesus said, the "very hairs of your head are all numbered." (Luke 12:7) We find more relationship to the lives we are leading, the work we are engaging in, and the aims and purposes we hold dear when we can see something working in the life of another person and changing it for the better. For this reason, I have endeavored to narrate in a brief form—but which, I hope, holds to an essential accuracy—a selected number of those cases which are listed in a chronological and skeletal fashion in the Appendix, Table V.

Case No. 12. A twenty-five-year old housewife, two-and-a-half months pregnant, was seen in our office on October 10, 1962, just twenty-four hours after she noted the onset of vaginal bleeding. The bleeding had stopped during the night, but a deep ache in the pelvic region persisted. She had just recovered two weeks prior from an acute upper respiratory infection. Examination, the first since the beginning of her pregnancy, showed a normal blood pressure of 100/60, temperature of 99 degrees, and pelvic findings of early pregnancy, including an enlarged uterus and a cervix which was soft and bluish. Her last menstrual period was July 25, 1962. Diagnosis was early pregnancy with threatened abortion.

As treatment, the patient was instructed to stay at bed rest for the next three days, to use castor oil packs on the low abdomen for one hour three times a day for one week, then three times a week for four weeks.

Follow-up revealed disappearance of the ache in the pelvic region within the next three days and no recurrence of the bleeding throughout the pregnancy, which terminated normally at nine months.

Response was rated as excellent to single therapy.

Case No. 33. An eighty-nine-year-old retired teacher with a delightful sense of humor developed severe abdominal distention. This distention had begun two weeks prior to that time and was shortly followed by nausea and vomiting. The latter became more severe and gradually more foul-smelling. There was no fever, but discomfort developed into pain in the abdomen.

She had a history of two other episodes of this nature. One occurred four years prior to the present illness, wherein she was hospitalized and decompressed with a Miller-Abbott tube, saline enemas, and cathartics. (The second is part of this series as Case No. 32. She had responded well two years before to the use of castor oil packs on this occasion.) Physical findings upon examination revealed a plus-three ankle edema, marked abdominal distention with drum-like stretching of the skin of the abdomen, and active peristalsis with frequent peristaltic rushes. She had not had a good bowel movement in "a long time." She had taken a mild laxative several times before calling me to her home. Diagnosis was intestinal obstruction due to fecal impaction.

Therapy consisted of diet and castor oil packs. She was placed on nothing by mouth except ice chips for forty-eight hours. The packs were begun immediately—without the use of the heating pad as normally instructed—and they were continued without interruption for six full days. As soon as the packs were started, all the symptoms eased up and the vomiting slowed down. An evacuant rectal suppository was used after forty-eight hours, with good returns, and the vomiting stopped. Distention rapidly disappeared and, at the end of the six days, the belly was flat, the ankle edema had been completely relieved, and the patient was having normal bowel movements, telling jokes and watching television again. The family reported her in "remarkable" condition. Her diet by this time was back to normal.

Response was rated as excellent to single therapy.

Case No. 42. A sixty-five-year-old housewife was seen initially within several hours of the onset of severe right upper quadrant pain, nausea, and vomiting, following the ingestion of a heavy meal the prior evening. She gave a history of having had hypertension for some time and of being overweight, but no past history of gall bladder disease. Examination revealed tenderness over the area of the gall bladder. There was no mass palpable, but there was question of increased dullness to percussion in the area where the gall bladder lies. Blood pressure was 142/86. Temperature was normal. Body weight 166 pounds. The diagnosis was acute cholecystitis (inflammation of the gall bladder).

Food was withheld until nausea left. The only therapy used was castor oil packs, applied all night long each night for six nights. The vomiting stopped the first night. Pain was "fifty percent less" the following morning, then gradually subsided. Examination on the sixth day showed the absence of any tenderness. Two pain pills were used during the first day of therapy. On the evening of the fourth, fifth, and sixth days of therapy, the patient was instructed to take one ounce of olive oil by mouth.

Response was rated as excellent to single therapy.

Case No. 44. A sixty-two-year-old retired carpenter injured his right index finger twenty-four hours before coming to our office. He had run a splinter into the tissues of the dorsum of the finger near the nail, but he thought he had gotten all of it out. However, the next day, the finger was inflamed and very tender and he sought help. Examination showed a puncture wound of the dorso-medial aspect of the finger and, surrounding the puncture site, the tissues were acutely inflamed, causing moderate swelling of the entire distal end of the finger. A small incision was made, enlarging the wound, and a 5/8" intact wood splinter was removed, releasing one-half to one-and-a-half cc. of pus which had formed in the irritated area. Diagnosis was infected puncture wound of the right index finger.

A dressing was fashioned for the finger made of soft flannel cloth soaked in castor oil, around which was wrapped plastic, then a simple gauze dressing. This was allowed to remain in place for forty-eight hours. On examination at that point, all swelling, inflammation, and tenderness were absent and the incision healed. It should be noted here that usual response to removal of a foreign body that has caused a local cellulitis is rapid repair and healing, but it seldom is seen to respond this quickly with usual post-operative care.

Response thus was rated excellent to single therapy.

Case No. 58. A thirty-nine-year-old music teacher presented himself with the complaint of having had a right-sided headache for the past thirteen days. He had no prior history of such difficulty, and all measures he had taken had not produced any significant results. Examination revealed a normal blood pressure of 120/90. There was rather marked tenderness on palpation, but all other findings were well within normal limits. He had used salicylates and spasmolytics and had been given manipulative therapy to the upper spine and neck, but the headaches had persisted. Diagnosis was right-sided headache associated with right cervical muscular spasm.

The patient was instructed to use castor oil packs as a type of muffler around his neck, overlapping them onto his upper back toward the shoulders, and using the heating pad, adjusted so that it would be moderately hot. This, applied when he went to bed, was to be used most of each night. After two nights of treatment, the headache disappeared, and the patient discontinued the treatment. Examination on the seventh day showed absence of any tenderness in the previously described areas.

Response was rated excellent to single therapy.

Case No. 73. A twenty-one-year-old housewife who had wrestled with the problem of obesity (220 pounds) for several years presented herself in our office with the complaints of a sensation of pressure and gas in the lower abdomen when walking or being physically active in any way. The condition had persisted for a period of two to three weeks. She had had no serious illnesses in the past and had experienced no symptoms like these before this time. Examination revealed a normal blood pressure of 130/75 and the obesity described. Examination of the pelvis showed an ill-defined mass in the area of the right tube and ovary which was quite tender on palpation. Vagina and uterus were normal. There was no fever. Diagnosis was probably ovarian cyst, although it was difficult to rule out tubal pathology.

No therapy was used except castor oil packs, which were applied for one hour daily over the lower abdomen for a period of seven days.

Examination after the seven days of therapy revealed that the sensation of a mass was still present but considerably smaller, and the tenderness was lessened to a similar degree. The patient stated that all pain in the lower abdomen had disappeared with therapy continuing. Still later examination revealed that all signs of the mass had disappeared.

Response was rated excellent to single therapy. (A postscript to this case history is in order. This same woman returned still later for care for pregnancy, and it was determined that she must have been about two weeks pregnant when she was seen with the pain in the lower abdomen. What this means in reference to the signs and symptoms observed has not been determined at this writing.)

Perhaps the procedure of presenting six cases that were rated excellent in their response when no therapy other than the packs was utilized might be classified as putting one's right foot forward.

However, nonresponsive cases can be found in the Appendix, and I will comment on some of them.

There is another reason which prompted the use of these particular case reports. They represent a good cross section of how the packs are used most of the time and the general areas of the body that receive most attention from this oil from the Palma Christi.

There is something mysterious in the manner in which these applications of hot castor oil, soaked in flannel cloth and applied to the skin, bring about a sometimes startling change in the way the body is functioning. Even now it has caused me at times, while I watch what is going on with unbelieving eyes, to ask myself, "What happened?" What really goes on within the body that restores a disturbed gravid uterus to normal? That cures a muscular spasm and dissipates a headache? That allows an inflamed gall bladder to regain its health? That heals an infected wound? That gets rid of a threatening appendicitis as if it were no more than a mild cough? That mobilizes a fecal impaction which hours earlier had threatened a life? That rids the body of a disturbance in the reproductive system that might have dislodged a pregnancy before the mother even knew she was carrying a child? What happens when castor oil is applied, many times without any heat, that can have such an effect? How is it absorbed? Why does it work? *How* does it work?

These are questions whose answers are hard to come by. There are those who will say that they do not need answers because it has not been statistically proven that the packs work. The case reports, however, speak for themselves. Each tells a story. Almost routinely, the individual who uses a pack for the first time will change from a questioning, hesitant user to a happily surprised enthusiast. Thus it is my personal opinion that the questions expressed above do not need an answer, for we see something here that is working in the life of another person and changing it for the better.

Before we look more closely at a few of these cases to seek out some of the mechanisms which might be involved, it is well to investigate and comment on several different, more general aspects of the study.

Appendicitis assumes some degree of importance here since five cases are included among the eighty-one total forming the basis of the study. In looking at the ages, it is observed that they were ten, eleven, nine, forty-six, and ten years of age in that order. All the youngsters responded with exceeding promptness to therapy. One, Case No. 55, was given an antibiotic injection and a tranquilizer-antinausea suppository when seen, but overnight his nausea, lower abdominal cramping and pain, and his vomiting (all of three days' duration) were gone when he was examined the next morning, after using the packs all night. His abnormal tenderness was also absent and all findings were normal.

Two of the cases are reported at length elsewhere in the text or Appendix, but the fourth child, Case No. 9, is not. He noted onset of abdominal pain two days prior to his visit to my office, he vomited once and had some cramping pains in his belly. These symptoms eased up the next day somewhat, but recurred the following morning. There was no diarrhea, but some nausea. Examination showed a subnormal temperature of 97.8 degrees and well localized tenderness over the right lower quadrant. A slightly inflamed pharynx was also noted. The packs without heat were used three times a day for two days, when re-examination showed only minimal tenderness at the umbilicus (which subsequently cleared) and absence of the abdominal discomfort which the body had noted.

The question of the appendicitis as it occurred in the

adult, however, was another story. Nausea and lower abdominal pain had their onset at 2:30 p.m. and were thought to be due to food ingestion. The castor oil packs were kept on for about twelve hours, brought no relief, and the patient was hospitalized. A complicating renal infection was suspected but ruled out by intravenous pyelogram. Surgery for the appendix was decided upon when the tenderness became more localized and diagnostic. Thus we see in Case No. 37 that the response to this type of treatment was not adequate. The fact that there was a renal irritation complicated the picture, however, in this instance.

We find four excellent results, then; the only failure being in a middle-aged woman. If any inference were to be drawn from such a picture, it would be that the young people were much more able to muster the forces of resistance to disease on stimulation or to respond to a therapeutic measure with greater speed and efficiency.

There was no heat other than accumulated body heat involved in these particular cases. The oil was applied and certainly was absorbed to some extent. Perhaps these five cases point toward the concept that the castor oil, when absorbed, stimulates the bodily function that will remove the products of inflammation (as they exist in the appendix) from the appendix itself, leaving it freer to function normally. Under usual conditions the appendix, as all portions of the body, can handle irritations easily and maintain a condition of health. This is what is called natural body immunity; we see the story of the thymus, the lymphatic system, and natural immunity unfolding before us every day in these areas of research.

As has already been discussed, the functioning of the lymphatic system is closely allied with the normal function of the autonomic nervous system. The parasympathetic gives motor innervation to the lymphatics, wherever it has been shown to exist. The parasympathetic is also termed the system which brings rebuilding and healing to the body.

Earlier it was hypothesized that the lymphatics drain wastes from the individual cells much as the intestines remove wastes from the body. Thus we see the framework for a mechanism which could be effective in these four cases of appendicitis and which would even explain why one did not respond.

Castor oil absorbed into the tissues may, in its vibratory activity (for all things are in essence vibratory in nature), act to stimulate that parasympathetic nerve supply which is anatomically located in the area treated, which then would stimulate the lymphatics to drain more adequately the tissues under duress, perhaps at the same time acting directly on the lymphatics to perform the function just stated. Any organ or portion of the body which is clogged with waste products which the lymphatics have not removed would theoretically respond in a beneficial way to any procedure which would bring about an alleviation of that condition.

With such a mechanism in operation, it can be readily seen that anyone who has gone downhill relative to resistance, endurance, response to injury, or general body health would not have a topnotch thymus-lymphatic system—the basic regulator of health and disease. Such a person would have a slower response or perhaps little response at all to stimulation toward healing.

In looking at the other portion of such a healing mechanism, one can understand how healing would be a less dramatic process if the parasympathetic nervous system were under sufficient stress or tension that it would refuse to respond to the vibratory activity of the castor oil as it is absorbed into the tissues. The heat, when used, may just accentuate the basic reaction to the castor oil of the tissues involved. When heat could cause an adverse response within the body, of course, the benefits of this therapeutic measure are far outweighed by its detrimental effects.

Appendicitis, obstructions, and other similar conditions are among those in which heat is specifically contraindicated because of the complications which might be brought about by the increased vascularity and metabolic activity. In these, the only benefits obtained from use of the packs must come from the castor oil itself. How the oil brings about changes within the body is, at this point, not at all explored or understood.

In Case No. 33, different factors than one would usually find in appendicitis are at work. In this instance, there had been a large bowel impaction with fecal material that produced actual intestinal obstruction to the degree that serious consequences were already being experienced. The large bowel was probably nearing a point of complete inactivity insofar as its proper duties of evacuation were concerned, and the small bowel was so at war with events as they were transpiring that reverse peristalsis was bringing fecal material up to the stomach to be expelled through persistent episodes of emesis. Gas throughout the system producing serious distention completed the picture of an intestinal tract that had moved a long way from its original state of health to provide peristalsis and moisture sufficient to move the bowels regularly and without difficulty.

It should be recalled that the organs and structures of elimination—both the large bowel from the midpoint of the transverse colon on and the urinary system—receive their motor innervation from the parasympathetic portion of the autonomic nervous system which has its source in the sacral nerves of the body. This eighty-nine-year-old woman spent a lot of her time sitting and, with little padding on her buttocks, undoubtedly produced many pressures on the sacral portion of her anatomy which could easily, and probably did, cause embarrassment to the sacral nerve supply. Reinforced by poor bowel habits and a diet that was not perfect and enhanced by practically no exercise, the entire motor system of nerves to the large bowel undoubtedly became sluggish to the point of nearly complete inactivity.

Then packs were applied to the abdomen. Nausea ceased, emesis slowed down and stopped, peristalsis began in the large bowel, enough fluid was produced by the cells of the large bowel to soften the fecal mass, and the health of the cells throughout the intestinal cavity improved. After forty-eight hours, when an evacuant suppository was used, the intestine was in good enough health to respond normally and the contents were expelled. It is interesting to note also that the edema which had persisted then disappeared, undoubtedly due to the more efficient functioning of the other portion of the eliminating system, the kidneys.

Was the action here brought about through nerve tissue stimulation, or was it perhaps another instance where cells were cleansed and thus worked more normally? The answer, of course, remains hypothetical. The fact that she improved is evident. That she made a remarkable change physiologically cannot be denied. That she had no medication with which to do this—other than castor oil packs—is also factual. Still, the method of restoring her health is not yet clear.

One factor which has not been discussed relative to this particular patient is her sense of humor. She even handled pain with a joke and a smile. Her ability to keep the people who took care of her in good humor made the job easier for all concerned. The part that this attitude of joy and happiness plays in the continuance of good health has not yet been adequately evaluated, but it has to be a major factor wherever it exists. It is well known that ire at the dinner table brings about indigestion, while a happy meal is a beneficial one. Humor, then, must help the gastrointestinal tract, perhaps far more than we know or realize. In a similar manner, it may be that this little old lady is alive only because of her happy disposition. Whatever is true, she remains a favorite of mine.

The diagnosis of cholecystitis brings a different group of organs into consideration. It would be of interest and of value to our understanding to visualize, if possible, what must take place while an inflamed gall bladder is being restored to normal function. Cholecystitis may vary in severity from an acute catarrhal condition with congestion and edema to a condition of acute suppuration, wherein the walls of the gall bladder exude frank pus, and the peritoneal surface is covered by an acute exudate.

In Case No. 42, events had undoubtedly not progressed far enough to bring about the latter condition cited in the above paragraph. In all likelihood, the walls of the gall bladder were slightly inflamed and thickened with the congestion of blood and lymphatic vessels and with edema; the bile was probably thickened; the cystic duct leading out of the gall bladder toward the common duct was probably swollen shut with the same processes; and the gall bladder was probably distended with bile. There may have been a stone or many small stones obstructing the opening of the cystic duct, but this can sometimes only be determined at surgery if x-rays do not confirm the presence of stones.

Most likely there were conditions present as described, without the stones, and these conditions must be returned to normal by body processes in order to avoid the necessity of surgical intervention. The only factor physically which can bring about the alleviation of the edema and congestion in the common duct and the wall of the gall bladder is an increase in the blood supply associated with an increased drainage from these areas via the lymphatics and veins.

It doesn't particularly matter whether this comes about through improved parasympathetic nerve function or through lessening of the sympathetic supply, which could theoretically achieve the same result, or through direct relaxation of the lymphatic and venous vessel walls, allowing freer flow into the general circulation. What part does infection play in all this? It is well known that a marked increase in blood flow through a part of the body—and that means increased flow from such a part as well—will overcome infection most of the time without any assistance.

As the cells involved in this process just described are allowed to function more normally, then a condition of health will gradually be restored to the tissue of the gall bladder and the cystic duct. To what level of health they are restored probably depends on many factors already established by habits of diet, levels of hormones, and balances established among the functioning of the systems which are involved. It is certainly a hazardous undertaking to try to understand at a different level how the body may function, when there are so many unknowns to deal with and the probability of error in thought and in deduction creates so many potential pitfalls. In an effort to understand the working of this therapy used in this and other cases, however, it becomes a considered risk.

One woman, Case No. 42 (mentioned just a few paragraphs earlier), had a rather typical history of gall bladder disease, and her physical findings substantiated the history. Her response to the castor oil packs throughout the night was dramatic, although simple hot packs have been recommended for this condition for years. The use of these packs, plus liquid diet, bed rest, and simple sedatives usually result in rapid disappearance of symptoms. It would be difficult to estimate here with any degree of accuracy whether the castor oil contributed more than the heat to the response which was noted.

Following the indications and inferences of the information we have thus far accumulated, however, we would assume that it had an effect. The degree of effect is left in question. Further work with this medium of therapy obviously is needed to demonstrate the level of effectiveness which might be achieved. Further comments on cholecystitis will not be attempted, although the reader can refer to the earlier portion of this book, where several of the Cayce readings touched on the same disease process.

Looking again at these case histories, we see that these two young ladies who became cases No. 12 and No. 73 had one thing in common: both were pregnant at the time they were treated with the packs. One was threatening to abort, while the other had a pelvic mass and did not know she was pregnant.

The packs, used conservatively not all night long as in several other cases—produced clinical evidence of improved function of the generative organs and their associated structures. At the same time, it became evident that through this medium of therapy, the body as a unit became more able to muster its defense mechanisms and reverse the conditions of ill health which were found to be present on initial examination. This area of the body—the uterus, vagina, and ovaries—where a woman becomes creative at least in the physical sense—is also the area where cleansing of the body takes place through excretion, as has been already noted earlier. The parasympathetic supply to both functions arises in the sacral nerves. So we wonder if these two functions—creativity and cleansing—don't have a closer association than we usually suspect. Would it be unrealistic to propose that any striving of humankind, when it is done with true creativity, is cleansing to the consciousness of the individual?

On the other hand, would it be more proper to state that any work or daily activity that a person might be faced with is done creatively in the truest sense if he or she feels a cleansing or a purification in consciousness? Bodily functions running parallel with so-called mental or spiritual values—these must be related to each other in the human being, if any of the philosophic, psychologic, religious, or theological concepts of the oneness of all things holds true validity. But this is perhaps philosophy in itself.

To return to the gynecological conditions under consideration, we may be seeing here the acceleration of cleansing as it occurs in the body, added to the stimulation of the creative or generative organs through the mechanism of the improved functioning of the sacral parasympathetic and its ramifications throughout the lower portion of the body. For this one source of activity the sacral parasympathetic would at least to some degree control the rebuilding forces within these organs and structures: the general eliminative activity and health of the body and the lymphatic activity as it pertains to drainage from cellular components within the area. These concepts have been more fully discussed elsewhere, but they are seen acting here within the human body to bring about health and its more desirable state of the body.

In considering that both these young women were pregnant, and that the effect on both pregnancies must certainly have been beneficial, one wonders how many birth abnormalities and anomalies might be prevented through use of a series of packs during early pregnancy as a preventative routine. If the activity of the packs is such as to improve function, as seems apparent, then it would follow rather naturally that less abnormal function would be found in the presence of more normal function. But then, perhaps it is not advisable nor permissible to be so direct in one's logic (a right use of thought or the rational powers). Or, perhaps more correctly, logic applied to an assumption remains an assumption. Whatever the case in regard to absolutely accurate use of the mind through steps which must be proved, it would still seem reasonable that one could, through the castor oil packs being used preventively, bring healthier babies into the world.

The two remaining cases, among those I selected to comment upon, have to do with use of the packs locally and in areas removed from body cavities. The music teacher, Case No. 58, used heat with the pack he applied to his neck and upper back and, within two days, the pain and headache of thirteen days' duration had disappeared. The mechanism here of relaxation of muscular cramping and spasm is certainly well understood at the present time. Other modes of therapy, including physiotherapy, might well have brought just as good results, but it is interesting that he had already used many other means of treatment with poor results when the packs were begun. My experience with other similar cases outside the present series (including myself as one of the prime examples), leads me to my present firm opinion and clinical position that this method of treatment becomes the treatment of choice in this particular group of conditions where muscular spasm is the primary pathology.

The heat is not the answer to the relaxation, else heat by itself would bring just as much response. It doesn't. But it is also questionable that the pack without the heat would do as well. The combination of the castor oil and the heat seems to bring about a more substantial therapeutic effect. As will be seen in the next case, that of the injured finger, the castor oil apparently brings about a specific response without the use of heat, and this is in body tissues where organs are not concerned. Here we find only skin, subcutaneous tissue, muscle, fascia, fat, interstitial tissue, blood vessels, nerves, lymphatics, and bone. There are no organs, no glands, no tubular structures, no lymph centers, and no ganglia or other nerve centers. We are again led to the conclusion that the castor oil, when absorbed, directs its activities in an exquisitely minute relationship to the tissues it contacts and stimulates those tissues afflicted toward a healthier function. It becomes difficult to deviate far from a concept that the cleansing or purifying of the individual cells affected is brought about through the medium of the lymphatics as related, at least in part, to the autonomic nerve supply to the area.

Case No. 44, the sixty-two-year-old man already referred to in the previous paragraph, presents really a rather remarkable story. Fingers such as his which have been infected and which have developed a pustular reaction so severe as to cause a rather diffuse cellulitis, simply do not very often clear up entirely in two days under the very best of therapeutic circumstances. This case, however, is somewhat representative of others which needed care in a postoperative or post-injury situation, such as those (Nos. 13, 14, 54, 65, 71, 74, and 76) in "Selected Cases." All of these people show how local tissues respond to the packs when injury or infection is present. The results are interesting and follow a certain pattern that has already been discussed.

Thus, we find the various areas where the packs can be used beneficially, the manner in which they may be used, and the type of response which may be seen are fairly well represented in the comments to this point.

Appendix

Notes About This Appendix

TABLE II IS A COMPILATION OF ALL THE diagnoses which were arrived at in the eighty-one cases which are being presented. Table III gives a breakdown of the types of illness treated and their response as a group. These are grouped together, as they seem to be relevant to this study rather than according to systems specifically or otherwise.

In Table IV can be found the most common conditions which were treated and how they responded.

Table V is a listing of all eighty-one cases showing identification, age, sex, diagnosis, and response to therapy.

From the information in this Appendix, it is seen that 74 of the 101 conditions responded in such a manner that they were rated in response as "excellent." This gives a healthy flavor to the results. It is fortunate that the human body takes even the least assistance at times and responds in a noble fashion. Even taking the assist of the unconscious vital forces of the body into consideration, the responses, especially in the group treated only with the packs, are highly gratifying.

When analyzing the information, one notes that there are no treatments for cardiac conditions, respiratory illnesses, basic neurological diseases (in spite of the important part this system plays in health and disease), or true endocrine difficulties (except those associated with the ovary and its function as seen in the diseases of the female generative system listed).

There are present, however, muscular conditions, arthritic disturbances, and systems problems with gastrointestinal, genitourinary, circulatory as it involves hypertension, and neurological as it involves headaches and tension syndromes. Trauma is also represented.

By far, the most common area treated anatomically is the abdomen and that which lies within the abdominal and pelvic cavities, the gastrointestinal, and the genitourinary systems. These make up well over fifty percent of the conditions treated. It would be helpful to recall at this point that Cayce speaks of the importance of the assimilation of foodstuffs into our bodies and the elimination of body wastes, and there is reference to castor oil packs being of benefit to both these systems. The kidneys, stomach, intestines, and their associated organs are the major areas of assimilation and elimination in the body. Thus, we would expect these areas to show beneficial response to the packs, if information from the readings were to have significance in clinical trial.

From Table III we see that there were a total of thirty treated conditions which have their site of pathology in the abdominal cavity or pelvis and which were treated with castor oil packs only. Results obtained were twenty-five excellent—eighty-three percent—two good, and three poor. This is slightly better than the percentage found in the entire series when this mode of therapy was used by itself.

Diseases of the large bowel produced the highest percentage of excellent response—ninety-two percent—these including such conditions as constipation, intestinal obstruction due to fecal impaction, colitis, diarrhea, hemorrhoids, and rectal fissures.

Interestingly, the two conditions which were most refractive to treatment in this series were essential hypertension and peptic ulcer (see Table IV). The two which produced the most consistently excellent results were those conditions found under traumatically induced conditions and post-surgical care of wounds. All twelve of these responded promptly and were rated as excellent. Only two of the twelve were given therapy other than the packs.

TABLE I

Number of Cases Surveyed	81
Number of Different Diagnoses	52
Total Conditions Treated	101
Treated with Castor Oil Packs Only	57
Excellent Results	47% - 82%
Good Results	4% - 7%
Poor Results	6% - 11%
Treated with Combined Therapy*	44
Excellent Results	27% - 61%
Good Results	3% - 7%
Poor Results	14% - 32%

*Combined therapy is the use of castor oil packs associated with other therapies that may have influenced the outcome of the condition.

CLASSIFICATION OF RESULTS

Excellent: Those cases in which response was prompt, as evaluated clinically, and complete—that is, progressing to expected end point and having no residual signs or symptoms of presenting condition.

Good: Those cases in which response was slower than expected; and/or whose presenting signs and symptoms did not completely disappear at the end point of therapy.

Poor: Those cases which showed no response to therapy, or which worsened under treatment given, or in which signs and symptoms did not materially change.

TABLE II
LIST OF DIAGNOSES

Abscess	Trichomoniasis	Peptic Ulcers
Abdominal Tenderness	Menopausal Syndrome	Constipation
Essential Hypertension	Mastitis (in male)	Appendicitis
Subpatellar Bursitis	Gastritis	Endometritis
Cholecystitis	Acute Cervical Sprain	Sprain of L. Biceps
Intestinal Obstruction	Salpingitis	Uterine Fibroid
Ovarian Cyst	Pyelonephritis	Diarrhea
Cystitis	Cervicitis	Colitis
Low Back Pain	Uterine Inertia	Infectious Hepatitis
Furuncle	Verruca Vulgaris	Threatened Abortion
Tinea Corporis, Perineum	Osteoarthritis	Fibrohematoma
Menorrhagia	Rectal Fissure	Hemoperitoneum
Peritoneal Adhesions	Cellulitis of Axilla	Hemorrhoids
Sebaceous Cyst	Vaginitis	Tenosynovitis
Purpura, Traumatic	Oophoritis	Bursitis of Shoulder
Hematoma, Subungual	Headache, Myositis	Tension Syndrome
Abrasions, Lacerations	Infected Puncture Wound	Oral Contraceptive Reaction

TABLE III		Packs Only			Combined		
TYPES AND NUMBER OF CONDITIONS TREATED AND RESPONSES		Excellent	Good	Poor	Excellent	Good	Poor
Diseases of the Female Generative System	22	7	0	1	12	0	2
Diseases of the Lower Bowel	15	11	0	1	1	1	1
Diseases of the Upper Digestive Tract, Liver, and Gall Bladder	11	2	1	0	3	0	5
Appendicitis	5	3	0	1	1	0	0
Abdominal Tenderness, Undiagnosed	2	2	0	0	0	0	0
Postoperative Peritoneal Adhesions	1	0	1	0	0	0	0
Diseases of the Urinary Tract	4	0	0	0	4	0	0
Headaches and Tension Syndromes	5	2	0	0	2	1	0
Essential Hypertension	5	0	0	0	1	0	4
Local Infections	11	6	1	0	1	1	2
Traumatically Induced Conditions	7	6	0	0	1	0	0
Post-Surgical Care	5	4	0	0	1	0	0
Sebaceous Cysts	2	1	0	1	0	0	0
Arthritic Conditions	6	3	1	2	0	0	0
Total:	101	47	4	6	27	3	14

Number of conditions treated with abdominal packs   61

Number of conditions treated with localized packs   50

MOST COMMON CONDITIONS TREATED AND RESPONSE		Packs Only			Combined		
		Excellent	Good	Poor	Excellent	Good	Poor
Abscess	6	4	1	0	1	0	0
Hypertension	5	0	0	0	1	0	4
Hemorrhoids	6	5	0	1	0	0	0
Appendicitis	5	3	0	1	1	0	0
Infected Puncture Wounds	4	3	0	0	1	0	0
Duodenal Ulcer— Peptic Ulcer	4	0	0	0	1	0	3
Total:	30	15	1	2	5	0	7

TABLE IV

Number of conditions treated with abdominal packs   61
Number of conditions treated with localized packs   50

TABLE V: RESPONSE TO THERAPY

Case No.	Case Diagnosis	Castor Oil Packs Only			Combined Rx		
		Ex-cellent	Good	Poor	Ex-cellent	Good	Poor
1	M. 53 Yrs. Abscess of Buttocks	x					
2	F. 46 Yrs. Trichomoniases				x		
3	M. 44 Yrs. Duodenal Ulcer						x
4	F. 47 Yrs. Gastritis				x		
	Tension Syndrome				x		
	Menopausal Syndrome				x		
	Slight Vascular Hypertension				x		
5	M. 24 Yrs. Mastitis, Left Breast						x
6	F. 39 Yrs. Cervicitis				x		
	Right Oophoritis				x		
	Endometritis, Chronic, Mild				x		
7	F. 13 Yrs. Left Subpatellar Bursitis	x					
8	M. 33 Yrs. Constipation, Chronic	x					
	Cholecystitis, Chronic	x					
9	M. 10 Yrs. Appendicitis	x					
10	M. 43 Yrs. Duodenal Ulcer				x		
11	F. 58 Yrs. Diarrhea				x		
12	F. 25 Yrs. Threatened Abortion	x					
13	F. 75 Yrs. Abscess, Left Axilla	x					
14	M. 11 Yrs. Fibrohematoma of Subcutaneous Tissue	x					
15	M. 37 Yrs. Cystitis				x		
	Pyelonephritis				x		
16	F. 51 Yrs. Colitis, Mucus					x	

TABLE V: RESPONSE TO THERAPY

Case No.	Case Diagnosis	Castor Oil Packs Only			Combined Rx		
		Ex-cellent	Good	Poor	Ex-cellent	Good	Poor
17	F. 32 Yrs. Cervical Erosion (Cervicitis)	x					
	Uterine Fibroid?			x			
18	M. 11 Yrs. Appendicitis	x					
19	F. 29 Yrs. Cervicitis				x		
	Salpingitis				x		
20	M. 66 Yrs. Gastritis						x
21	F. 51 Yrs. Constipation	x					
	Headache, Chronic					x	
	Vaginitis				x		
22	F. 16 Yrs. Low Back Pain	x					
23	F. 32 Yrs. Uterine Inertia, Post Partum				x		
24	F. 42 Yrs. Hemorrhoids	x					
25	M. 32 Yrs. Abscess, Perirectal Tissues	x					
27	M. 9 Yrs. Appendicitis	x					
28	M. 11 Yrs. Hepatitis, Infectious		x				
29	M. 69 Yrs. Furuncle (Post- I & D)	x					
30	F. 40 Yrs. Verruca Vulgaris	x					
31	F. 19 Yrs. Hemoperitoneum	x					
32	F. 86 Yrs. Intestinal Obstruction (Fecal)	x					
33	F. 89 Yrs. Intestinal Obstruction (Fecal)	x					

TABLE V: RESPONSE TO THERAPY

Case No.	Case Diagnosis	Castor Oil Packs Only			Combined Rx		
		Ex-cellent	Good	Poor	Ex-cellent	Good	Poor
34	F. 54 Yrs. Tinea Corporis, Perineum				x		
35	F. 20 Yrs. Pyelonephritis				x		
	Threatened Abortion				x		
36	F. 42 Yrs. Oral Contraceptive Reaction	x					
	Hypertension						x
37	F. 46 Yrs. Appendicitis			x			
38	M. 33 Yrs. Rectal Fissures	x					
39	F. 70 Yrs. Abdominal Tenderness (No Dx.)	x					
40	F. 58 Yrs. Multiple Small Lacerations with Swelling of Tissues, Left Knee	x					
41	F. 72 Yrs. Colitis	x					
	Tension Syndrome				x		
	Hypertension						x
42	F. 65 Yrs. Cholecystitis	x					
43	F. 62 Yrs. Abdominal Tenderness (Etiology?)	x					
44	M. 62 Yrs. Infected Puncture Wound, Left Index Finger	x					
45	M. 50 Yrs. Hemorrhoids			x			
46	F. 47 Yrs. Cellulitis, Left Axilla	x					

TABLE V: RESPONSE TO THERAPY

Case No.	Case Diagnosis	Castor Oil Packs Only			Combined Rx		
		Ex-cellent	Good	Poor	Ex-cellent	Good	Poor
47	M. 64 Yrs.						
	Ulcer, Gastro-duodenal Penetrating with Pyloric Stenosis						x
	Ulcer, Anterior						x
	Cholecystitis, Chronic						x
48	F. 45 Yrs.						
	Sebaceous Cyst			x			
49	F. 40 Yrs.						
	Gastritis and Duodenitis				x		
50	F. 67 Yrs.						
	Hypertension						x
51	F. 38 Yrs.						
	Menorrhagia						x
	Uterine Fibroid						x
52	F. 53 Yrs.						
	Tension Syndrome	x					
	Vaginitis				x		
53	M. 10 Yrs.						
	Infected Puncture Wound (Left Foot)				x		
54	F. 54 Yrs.						
	Purpura, Traumatic in Origin	x					
55	M. 10 Yrs.						
	Appendicitis				x		
56	F. 45 Yrs.						
	Peritoneal Adhesions, Nonsymptomatic			x(?)			
57	M. 37 Yrs.						
	Tenosynovitis, Right Foot				x		
58	M. 39 Yrs.						
	Headache	x					
	Myositis, Right Cervical	x					
59	M. 17 Yrs.						
	Abscess, Left Calf	x					
60	F. 59 Yrs.						
	Hypertension, Essential						x

TABLE V: RESPONSE TO THERAPY

Case No.	Case Diagnosis	Castor Oil Packs Only			Combined Rx		
		Ex-cellent	Good	Poor	Ex-cellent	Good	Poor
61	F. 51 Yrs. Menopausal Syndrome	x					
62	F. 17 Yrs. Cellulitis, Left Axilla						x
63	F. 41 Yrs. Endometritis, Chronic, Low Grade					x	
64	F. 56 Yrs. Hemorrhoids	x					
65	M. 25 Yrs. Infected Puncture Wound	x					
66	F. 25 Yrs. Myositis, Left Trapezius Group	x					
67	F. 52 Yrs. Bursitis, Right Shoulder	x					
68	M. 64 Yrs. Sebaceous Cyst, Draining	x					
69	M. 53 Yrs. Hemorrhoids	x					
70	F. 40 Yrs. Colitis, Chronic Mucus						x
71	M. 5 Yrs. Contaminated Puncure Wound	x					
72	M. 60 Yrs. Abscess, Right Chest Wall					x	
73	F. 21 Yrs. Right Ovarian Cyst	x					
74	M. 64 Yrs. Hematoma, Subungual, Secondary to Fracture	x					
75	F. 62 Yrs. Cervical Sprain, Acute Trauma				x		
76	F. 17 Yrs. Sprain of Left Biceps, Radial Insertion	x					
77	F. 58 Yrs. Osteoarthritis, Cervical and Right Deltoid Area			x			

TABLE V: RESPONSE TO THERAPY

Case No.	Case Diagnosis	Castor Oil Packs Only			Combined Rx		
		Ex-cellent	Good	Poor	Ex-cellent	Good	Poor
78	M. 49 Yrs. Hemorrhoids	x					
79	M. 62 Yrs. Hemorrhoids	x					
80	F. 43 Yrs. Pyelonephritis, Acute				x		
81	F. 54 Yrs. Tenosynovitis, Left Foot			x			

Selected Cases

THIS PORTION OF THE APPENDIX IS A GROUP of narrative summaries of a selected group of cases that are, in my opinion, of the most interest to the reader. These summaries are in addition to the cases that have already been cited.

The emotions, responses within the individual to conditions outside the body in relationship to other people and self's evaluation of self, bring about within the body a disturbance that often sees certain areas affected according to the emotions' experiences. But the balance within the body organs and body systems becomes disturbed, elimination is hindered, intake of food is associated with turmoil, and the beginnings of body sickness are seen through just the mechanisms which here have been only lightly touched upon.

The circulatory system to various parts of the body, as it is related to the autonomic, is a site of disturbance frequently mentioned. These relationships were not made clear in the study reported on here nor were those which bring together the efficacy of the castor oil packs in pelvic diseases and the sacral parasympathetic supply to these organs.

Much in the way of psychologic function, as seen by the Cayce readings, becomes more understandable as serious study is given portions of the readings. The rationale of castor oil pack therapy begins to become apparent. Few, if any, contradictions show up in the startling number of words which flowed in such a strange manner from these lips of a dedicated man and the reaches of an unconscious mind.

We begin to see that it is not so strange that a castor oil pack can be applied to the abdomen and, in one person, a vaginitis is cleared up; in a second case, a fecal impaction causing intestinal obstruction is relieved; in a third, a threatened abortion is rendered into a normal pregnancy; in a fourth, a cholecystitis is cured; and in a fifth, after ten long months, the hair is made to suds and curl once more. Unless physiological factors that we do not wholly understand were at work, these things could not have occurred.

Cayce, whose work on these readings ceased in 1944 just prior to his death, would undoubtedly agree that this last readings extract would speak to these strange results from a strange therapy:

> For, what is the source of all healing for human ills? From whence doth the body receive life, light, or immortality? That the body as an active force is the result of spirit and mind, these coordinating and cooperating, enables the entity to bring forth in the experience that which may be used—or the using of the abilities of whatever nature. Each soul has within its power that to use which may make it at one with Creative Forces or God. These are the sources from which life, light, and the activity of body, mind and soul may manifest in whatever may be the active source or principle in

the mind of the individual entity . . .

There are, then, as given those influences in the nature of man that may supply that needed. For, man in his nature—physical, mental and spiritual—is a replica, is a part of whole universal reaction in materiality.

Hence there are those elements which if applied in a material way, if there is the activity with same of the spirit and mind, may bring into the experience of each atom of the body force or cell itself the awareness of the Creative Force or God. It may only rise as high as the ideal held by the body-mind.

Hence there is the one way, the source. For in Him is all life, all health, all mind, all knowledge and immortality to the soul-mind itself. (3492-1)

A PARTIAL LIST OF
RESEARCH CASES

Case No. 2. A forty-six-year-old housewife was seen with symptoms of pelvic discharge, urinary irritation, and low abdominal pain, which had persisted chronically for a period of at least three years. She was constantly under much strain as the result of marital tension. Examination showed tenderness over the uterus and in the area of the tubes and ovaries, and a heavy, yellowish vaginal discharge. She had been given a course of ten days' treatment using specific oral trichomonicidal tablets and vaginal suppositories with no adequate clearing of the condition. Her diagnosis was trichomoniasis.

She was instructed to again use the tablets, but no suppositories. She was started on castor oil packs placed on her lower abdomen for a one-hour period three times a week. She used the tablets for ten days and the packs for about two weeks. Her symptoms disappeared. She did not return for examination. Eight months later, the symptoms recurred. She medicated herself and took the packs once again. Her symptoms again subsided. The discharge did not recur. When she was examined eight months after that, the cervix was clean, there was no tenderness of the uterus (which was normal in size), and no discharge was found. She stated at that time that she had had occasional recurrence of mild lower abdominal soreness, for which she used the packs and relieved the soreness.

This case was evaluated as excellent response to combined therapy.

Case No. 3. A forty-four-year-old mechanical engineer was first seen with a two-week history of epigastric distress. He had a four-year history of bleeding peptic ulcer, but the last episode was treated with no bleeding being experienced. He had been medicating himself with an antacid. His examination showed a blood pressure of 135/80 and tenderness over the epigastric region and transverse colon area. Other findings were normal. His diagnosis was recurrent acute peptic ulcer.

He was started on specific antispasmodic and antacid therapy concurrently with the use of castor oil packs, which were given daily for one hour. Within twenty-four hours after being seen the first time and after one application of the packs, he started bleeding severely from the ulcer and was hospitalized. Bleeding was controlled in the hospital, diagnosis was confirmed by x-ray, and after discharge he was given a course of packs at home. These produced no appreciable response objectively or subjectively, so were discontinued.

Rating in this case was poor with combined therapy.

Case No. 7. A thirteen-year-old schoolgirl had fallen and injured her left knee the day before being seen in our office. The patella had been dislocated laterally, but had been reduced later. Examination showed much tenderness and subpatellar swelling. There were no fractures. Diagnosis was left subpatellar traumatic bursitis.

Treatment consisted only of castor oil packs, adminis-
tered for a half hour four times daily for the next five days.
The cooperation was excellent, the pain and swelling subsided rapidly, ambulation was encouraged from the
beginning, and when the patient was seen five days after
beginning of therapy, the swelling and tenderness were
gone and the patient asymptomatic.

Response rated excellent, using packs only.

Case No. 8.   A thirty-three-year-old male accountant
presented himself with the chief complaint of severe constipation for one month associated with generalized
abdominal distention. He gave a history of having had some
degree of chronic constipation with distention since childhood. During the month just past, he noted that laxatives
caused cramping and gave him no real relief. Examination
showed all findings to be within normal limits except for
abdominal tenderness, most marked over both lower quad-
rants. There was no tenderness noted over the gall bladder
area or the pancreas. He had been treated in the past with
contact evacuants, peristaltic stimulants, and cholagogue-
pancreatic enzyme mixture. The diagnosis used here is
constipation. The history is suspicious of pancreatic or
liver-gall bladder malfunction. A full work-up with x-ray
and laboratory tests was not performed.

Treatment consisted only of castor oil packs in association with a low-fat diet. The patient cooperated well in
applying the packs three days in a row each week for one
hour each time for a total of seven weeks. Results were very
satisfactory. The bowel movements became regular, the
cramps disappeared, and the abdominal pain ceased. Examination showed a normal abdomen with no tenderness
elicited.

Response rated as excellent to single therapy.

Case No. 13.   This seventy-five-year-old widow was a

resident of a rest home and was seen because of a boil which had developed in the left axilla. She complained of much pain associated with the furuncle, which was not draining. She had been hospitalized many times, once within the year earlier for surgical drainage of a furuncle in the right axilla. General health was poor and she had been an arthritic for many years. Examination of the local area showed much inflammation and swelling in the tissues of the boil and surrounding it. The patient complained of the pain and was unable to move her arm without much difficulty. No fluctuation could be found at that point. Diagnosis was furuncle of the left axilla.

No treatment was used except the castor oil packs twice daily for one-and-a-half hours for a period of seventeen days. The tenderness and pain subsided within the next two to three days and the furuncle gradually cleared until it disappeared completely. There was no evidence of fluctuation having occurred at any time, although the degree of tissue inflammation may have masked some of the signs which might otherwise have been observed. Thus there was no external drainage of material from this lesion at any time.

Response was rated as excellent to single therapy.

Case No. 14. This was an eleven-year-old boy who liked to play baseball. He was struck by a batted ball over the right maxilla (upper jawbone) two weeks before being seen in my office. The lump which developed in that area persisted and was gradually growing larger. Examination revealed an eight mm. fibrous tumor of the subcutaneous tissue overlying the right maxillary prominence, which was tender to palpation. X-rays were negative for fracture. Diagnosis was fibrohematoma of the subcutaneous tissues.

Treatment suggested was use of a castor oil pack to that area for forty-five minutes daily, to be used for a period of two weeks. The family cooperated very well and reported that the tenderness subsided in the first few days. The size of the nodule gradually became smaller. When he was examined in two weeks, the tumor was difficult to find because of its size, which was then perhaps two mm. in diameter and its consistency was softer. Treatment was stopped, and the nodule disappeared over a period of time.

Response was rated as excellent to single therapy.

Case No. 15. A thirty-seven-year-old male, married grocer, developed a urinary infection three days before being seen in our office on July 1, 1965. Symptoms were low back pain and urinary difficulty. His past history revealed two episodes of renal calculus in 1959 and 1963 and occasional upper respiratory infections. Examination showed tenderness over both costovertebral angles. Urinalysis showed albumen and the centrifuged specimen to be loaded with white blood cells. The patient was given a sulfa-azo dye medication and the infection cleared within a week, when the medication was stopped. Infection recurred two days later, but ten days' treatment did not now do the job, and the patient was seen on July 19, 1965, with original presenting symptoms. Diagnosis was cystitis and pyelonephritis.

Treatment with castor oil packs was begun on July 19, 1965, while continuing the other therapy. The packs were used over the renal areas of the low back all night for five nights. The aching subsided after the first night, recurred briefly on the third day, and then disappeared again. Examination on the fifth day showed absence of tenderness over the left costovertebral angle and only minimal tenderness over the right. The medication was cut to half dosage and the packs were continued to complete clearing of signs, symptoms, and laboratory evidence of infection.

Response was rated as excellent to combined therapy.

Case No. 16. A fifty-one-year-old housewife was in the midst of marital difficulties, which had progressed to divorce proceedings, when she was seen in our office with specific complaints of depression, nervousness, episodes of numbness, anorexia, nausea, abdominal cramps, and distention associated with much mucus in her stools that were loose in character. These had existed over a period of about two months, although she gave the history of having had symptoms of colitis over the past five-year period. Her physical examination showed a normal blood pressure of 100/70 and local findings of generalized abdominal tenderness, most marked in the epigastrium. There was hyperperistalsis present. Diagnosis for this survey purpose was mucous colitis. It is evident that there was a great deal of stress, tension, and depression present, but this was not evaluated as was the colitis, so was not used as a diagnosis.

Treatment was already being used: a colitis diet and two types of tranquilizers plus an antispasmodic for smooth muscles. These were continued and castor oil packs were added to the regimen, used three times a week for one-and-a-half hours daily over a period of four weeks. During this period of time, the cramps subsided, mucus no longer appeared in her stools, and the bowel movements became more normal. Peristalsis decreased. The packs were discontinued and sometime later most of the symptoms recurred.

Response was rated as good to combined therapy.

Case No. 18. An eleven-year-old schoolboy experienced the onset of abdominal pain with low-grade fever and vomiting while visiting relatives in California. The physician consulted stated that he had symptoms of appendicitis, gave him an injection of penicillin, and advised the parents to go home immediately to seek further care. He was brought to my office the next day with the history that he had continued to have nausea, anorexia, and abdominal pain. His temperature at that point was 98.6 degrees, and examination revealed tenderness in the right lower quadrant with positive rebound tenderness. There was no rigidity, no masses palpable, and peristalsis was present. Diagnosis was acute appendicitis.

The mother did not want surgery unless necessary. Since a critical point requiring surgical intervention had not arrived, I elected to watch and wait, instituting the use of castor oil packs without the use of the heating pad. The patient was put at bed rest, given only ice chips by mouth, and, with the pack on continuously, he remained comfortable the remainder of that day. He spent a good night, feeling much better in the morning. At that point, his nausea disappeared. On examination, his tenderness was only minimal and the rebound phenomenon was gone. He was given a full liquid diet, bed rest was continued, and the packs were kept on continuously. On the second morning of this therapy, the patient was completely asymptomatic. The packs were used two to four hours that day and a light diet was prescribed. Although there were no symptoms and the boy was impatient to be completely active, he was given the packs twice on the third day for one hour each. At that point, his diet was normal and he resumed full activity with no further therapy.

Response was rated as excellent to single therapy.

Case No. 22. A young sixteen-year-old housewife was seen in the office complaining of a low back pain of one week's duration. There was no history of injury or infection anywhere in the body. Urinalysis and blood count were both normal. There was a past history of irregular menses associated with mild obesity, but no serious illnesses. Her last menstrual period had been two-and-a-half months prior to her visit. Examination showed no abnormal physical findings. There was no sign of pregnancy or abnormality of the uterus. Diagnosis was low back pain of undetermined etiology.

Treatment was simple castor oil packs applied over the low back from the low sacral to the high lumbar area for one hour each day for ten days. When the patient was checked, she had no further symptoms.

Response was rated as excellent to single therapy.

Case No. 30. This was a forty-year-old married secretary who was seen with common warts on her right index finger which had been present for several months. The largest was eight mm. in diameter. Diagnosis was verruca vulgaris, right index finger.

These were treated by applying a Band-Aid® to the warts on the finger, the bandage portion being first soaked in castor oil. This was worn continuously, being changed once or twice a day for a period of two months. At the end of that time, the warts had completely disappeared.

Response was rated as excellent to single therapy.

Case No. 31. This was a nineteen-year-old mother of two children, the youngest of whom was eighteen months old. She had been on a contraceptive medication since her last pregnancy. Her complaint was pain and discomfort in the lower abdomen for two weeks, and for the past twenty-four hours she had been experiencing nausea and diarrhea with increased abdominal discomfort. She had started to menstruate three days prior to her visit. Examination showed a temperature elevation to 99.6 degrees. There was tenderness over the pelvic area, particularly with associated generalized abdominal tenderness. There were no masses, no rebound tenderness, and the peristalsis was active. Pelvic exam was deferred because of menses. Diagnosis was hemoperitoneum (blood in the peritoneum), due either to hemorrhagic cyst of the ovary which was leaking or to reflux of menstrual blood through one of the tubes.

The patient was placed on a liquid diet and at bed rest. She was instructed to apply castor oil packs to her lower abdomen for one hour twice during the remainder of that day and three times the next day. She was seen two days after her initial visit. All pain, discomfort, nausea, and diarrhea had stopped and patient felt fine. Only minimal tenderness remained suprapubically on examination. She did not return for further examination.

Response was rated as excellent to single therapy.

Case No. 36.   This patient was a forty-two-year-old housewife and registered nurse. This is perhaps the most unusual case in the series, and I refer to it fondly as "the case of the curly hair." This very interesting woman presented herself with the request that I check her blood pressure. She stated she had hypertension, and she believed it was due to taking a contraceptive medication for a period of time and to much tension. Her blood pressure had been discovered first to be elevated less than six months before her visit to our office. Her chronological story began, however, some sixteen months before this first visit. At that point she started taking contraceptive pills, which she continued for a total of thirteen months.

After being on the medication two months, she became embroiled in a series of traumatic family events that involved her daughter and her boyfriend. These events culminated in their effect in July of the following year, some seven months later. Meanwhile, at four months on the medication she developed noticeably increased nervousness. At five months she experienced a twenty-one-hour uterine hemorrhage that was difficult to stop. At the six-month period, she noted cramps in both legs.

At the nine-month mark, when personal tension was at its height, she developed swelling of the left calf and the cramps in her legs became at times excruciating. She also noted that when she washed her hair, for the first time in her life she could not make her hair develop a suds. She changed shampoos three times with no effect. The beauty parlor met with the same results: no sudsing.

At that point it was noted that her blood pressure was elevated. Her legs continued to severely bother her and the veins in her legs were distended until, after thirteen months on the medication, she stopped it of her own accord. Her gynecologist did not believe that the medication was caus-ing her trouble, according to her account. When she stopped the medication, her veins became normal and the cramps in her legs stopped bothering her. However, her blood pressure remained elevated, she remained tense, her hair retained the remarkable non-sudsing quality, the tex-ture of her hair was poorer, and her hair would not curl as well as it did before all this started.

She then saw an internist who examined her thoroughly and could find nothing wrong except the elevated blood pressure, which he did not think was caused by tension or by the medication. It was within a few weeks after this that she came to our office. Examination revealed a blood pres-sure of 180/110 to 160/98 with no other abnormal findings. She did not tell me about the hair until later, so there were no notations made about this condition. She was treated for three months with conventional medication for hyper-tension, and the blood pressure remained constant, not responding. About six months after she had stopped her medication, she complained of palpitation and tenseness again, and I was ready to begin use of the packs. Her diag-nosis, recorded for purposes of this study, was hypertension and oral contraceptive reaction.

Therapy was continued with the hypertensive medica-tion. The only other therapy advised was abdominal castor oil packs applied three consecutive nights each week for three weeks in a row with a one-hour duration for each treatment. The third pack each week was to be followed by oral ingestion of one ounce of olive oil. The patient followed the instructions and reported, when she returned in three weeks, that after one week's treatment with the packs, her hair sudsed like it hadn't in nearly ten months and there was a marked improvement in its texture and in its curling quali-ties. The hair was curly again. She noted no other change in symptoms.

Response was rated excellent to single therapy for the oral contraceptive reaction; poor to combined therapy for the hypertension.

Case No. 39. A seventy-year-old housewife had been bothered with dizziness which apparently brought on an attack of syncope (brief loss of consciousness), the cause of which had not been discovered. Several weeks after this, she developed abdominal tenderness and pain for which she sought our help. Her physical findings showed blood pressure to be 140/70; there was no fever. There was generalized, moderately severe abdominal tenderness. Pelvic examination was not performed. Blood count and urinalysis were normal. These findings were made one week after onset of the pain. The tentative diagnosis was abdominal tenderness, etiology undetermined (which is not a diagnosis, of course, but is descriptive of her symptomatology).

She was placed on vitamins, continued on the diet she was using, and she applied castor oil packs to her entire abdomen twice daily for one hour each time for a period of twelve days. She improved rapidly during the first three days and examination after twelve days showed all tenderness to be gone.

Response was rated as excellent to single therapy.

Case No. 41. A seventy-two-year-old married female, who was an apartment owner, presented herself with symptoms of nervous tension, associated with sickness in the family, and some swelling of the lower extremities and upper abdominal pain, all of which began several weeks prior to that time. She had a past history of hypertension, but general good health. Examination revealed a blood pressure of 160/90, obesity, moderate edema of both lower extremities, and tenderness over the upper abdomen across the area of the transverse colon. Her diagnoses were colitis of the transverse colon, tension syndrome, and hypertension.

She was started on therapy with a tranquilizer and a diuretic-hypertensive medication which she took faithfully. She was also instructed to use castor oil packs on her upper abdomen one hour at a time, three times daily for two weeks. She did not use the packs for the first two days because she didn't think they would do anything and they took too long to apply. During this time, she noted no benefit from the other two medications. When I reinforced the suggestion to use the packs, she did follow directions. She noted much subjective improvement from the very first. She stated that she obtained so much relief from the first pack that she slept three hours with it in place. She was able to return to work after three days. The pain was completely gone at the end of the two-week period, at which point all tenderness in the abdomen was absent. Her tension eased as the other symptoms and the findings improved. Her blood pressure, however, did not respond to therapy.

Response was rated excellent to single therapy for the colitis, excellent to combined therapy for the tension syndrome, and poor to combined therapy for the hypertension. It should be noted here that the tranquilizer by itself failed to bring relief for the tension, which the packs accomplished when added to the established therapy.

Case No. 47. A sixty-four-year-old male laborer presented himself for treatment because of the progression of symptoms of pain in the abdomen, vomiting, and general upper abdominal irritation. He had an exceptionally long history of gastrointestinal complaints, ulcer as diagnosed by x-ray, and repeated unsuccessful attempts to control the symptoms and the illness which persisted in the stomach. Examination showed a normal blood pressure and no fever, but tenderness over the entire abdomen, most marked over the epigastric area. Peristalsis was hyperactive. He had been treated with antibiotics, tranquilizers, and anti-secretory-type medications. Diagnosis used for purposes of this study were those listed as postoperative diagnoses: posterior penetrating gastroduodenal ulcer plus anterior duodenal ulcer plus pyloric stenosis plus chronic cholecystitis.

Treatment at this point was aimed at continuing his prior medication and adding the castor oil packs. He was instructed to use the packs twice daily for one hour each time over a two-week period. The response was not adequate, and he was referred to a surgeon who operated on him successfully some seventeen days after the packs were begun.

Response was rated poor to combined therapy for all the conditions listed. (This tends to "weight" the statistics unduly toward the negative response. However, there are other cases which "weight" things equally in the other direction. This is not a highly important factor in a study where statistics are only relatively important.)

Case No. 50.   A sixty-seven-year-old housewife had been treated for an unknown number of years for high blood pressure before she presented herself for examination and treatment at our office. She had experienced an episode of cystitis three months prior to that time, and a follow-up I.V. pyelogram was negative for any pathology. She gave a history of having had chronic sinusitis and had been allergic to many things throughout her lifetime. She did not experience any untoward symptoms from her blood pressure, but wanted to see it lower.

She had been under therapy with several types of antihypertensive and diuretic medications until three months prior, when she developed cystitis. These medications were then stopped, and she had been given a mild tranquilizer which she was using at bedtime. She took no other medication. Examination showed general negative findings with the exception of a blood pressure of 170/90. Her diagnosis was essential hypertension.

Therapy was continued with the tranquilizer and she was instructed to use castor oil packs for an hour each of three consecutive nights every week for a period of two months.

When she was examined at the end of that period of time, it was disclosed that her use of the packs was inconsistent. Blood pressure at that time was still 170/90. Blood pressure one month later was 160/100; seven months after that, 140/100; and six months following that, 158/88.

Response was rated poor to combined therapy.

Case No. 54.   A fifty-four-year-old housewife dropped an outdoor grill on her left foot the day prior to her visit in our office. Overnight, the initial pain grew worse and the foot became discolored and swollen. The patient could walk only with difficulty. No fractures were present, but examination revealed a two-plus edema, with tenderness and purpuric discoloration and swelling over the dorsum of the foot. She had taken one fifteen-minute Epsom salt bath treatment to the extremity.

Treatment consisted of castor oil packs to the foot twice daily for one hour for the next four days. She was to use an elastic bandage on the foot during this time. Examination on the fourth day revealed absence of all tenderness, purpura nearly gone, and the swelling markedly decreased. She had no more pain in the foot and she could walk without limp or difficulty.

Response was rated excellent to single therapy.

Case No. 63.   A forty-one-year-old housewife was seen in our office with a complaint of heaviness in the pelvis and a somewhat increased vaginal discharge of several weeks' duration. She gave the history of surgery for a teratoma at age twenty and of passing a renal calculus three months prior to her present visit. She stated that she frequently had episodes of vaginal discharge, whitish in nature and not severe. Examination showed a normal blood pressure and temperature. Pelvic examination revealed a yellowish-white vaginal discharge to be present; the uterus was enlarged and boggy and tender on palpation. Diagnosis was chronic low-grade endometritis.

Hot sitz baths were suggested to be taken three times a week, at bedtime, for twenty to thirty minutes. On alternate nights, the patient was instructed to apply castor oil packs to her lower abdomen for a one-hour period before retiring. This was to be continued for a four-week period. Cooperation by the patient was excellent and the course of therapy was finished. She was seen at the end of the four weeks and all the sensation of heaviness and aching were gone. She no longer had the vaginal discharge. Examination confirmed this; it also showed the uterus to be still just slightly enlarged and slightly tender, but decreased in size and firm to palpation.

Response was rated excellent to combined therapy.

Case No. 65. A twenty-five-year-old electrician presented himself with complaints of pain in the right hand in the area of a puncture wound. Five days prior a sliver of steel, lodged in the lateral aspect of the palm of the right hand, had been removed. Pain began about three days after that. Examination of the hand revealed an infected puncture wound with an area eight mm. in diameter of surrounding cellulitis. Diagnosis was infected puncture wound of the right hand.

A soft flannel cloth soaked in castor oil was applied to the inflamed area after being folded once or twice. Then a plastic covering was placed over this and then an elastic bandage was used with light tension around the hand. The patient was instructed to leave it in place for seventy-two hours. When he was examined, all pain had stopped and the inflammation was gone. The puncture wound had healed completely and the patient was discharged. There was no recurrence. No other therapy was used.

Response was rated excellent to single therapy.

Case No. 68. A sixty-four-year-old railroad worker developed a swelling, associated with tenderness, behind his left ear which grew gradually worse until, after a week, he came to our office for treatment. Examination revealed that a sebaceous cyst which had become inflamed and infected had started to drain spontaneously. The adjacent tissues had also become inflamed.

Treatment was a local castor oil pack applied over the involved area behind the ear and instructions were to leave the pack on all night long every night. He was seen two days later, and all tenderness and inflammation were gone and no further treatment was needed.

Response was rated excellent to single therapy.

Case No. 71. A five-year-old boy, just about ready to start kindergarten, was playing barefoot outside his home when he ran across an old plank of wood and drove a four-inch-long sliver through the sole of his left foot. It broke off and was removed by his parents who brought him into our office. He was unable to put weight on his foot and complained of pain. Examination revealed a through and through stab wound on the plantar aspect of the left foot, with two puncture wounds identified. They were bleeding only minimally. Examination showed no foreign bodies remaining in the wound. Diagnosis was through and through puncture wound of left foot.

Aside from routine tetanus protection given to such injuries, the only therapy used was castor oil packs, which were applied over the entire plantar aspect of the left foot and used continuously—without the heating pad most of the time—for forty-eight hours. All pain subsided rapidly, the patient became completely ambulatory and complained of no difficulty of any sort, and the wounds needed no further care after the two days of treatment.

Response was rated excellent to single therapy.

Case No. 74. A sixty-four-year-old pool maintenance man dropped a sixty-seven-pound drum on the toes of his right foot. X-ray showed a fracture of the tuft of the great toe and a fracture of the distal phalanx of the second toe. There was much pain associated with the injury and any motion or pressure to either toe was painful. Examination showed swelling of both toes with redness and a subungual (under the nail) hematoma on the great toe. The nail was not removed because of the trauma and fracture already present. The tissues of the great toe were markedly injured with much swelling. Diagnosis was subungual hematoma secondary to fracture of tuft of great toe.

Treatment consisted of castor oil pack to the great toe and to the second toe twice daily for an hour and a half to be continued for two weeks. He was given a soft slipper to wear on the affected foot and told not to bear weight on it. The tenderness subsided rapidly; the hematoma was gone in seven days; the patient was wearing his own shoes in ten days, at which time all tenderness was gone; and he was discharged in fourteen days, asymptomatic and with all swelling and tenderness gone.

Response was rated excellent to single therapy.

Case No. 76. A seventeen-year-old female high school senior was seen in the office complaining of pain in her left arm as a result of injuring it during physical education class earlier that day. She explained that she was doing pull-ups when she suddenly experienced a sharp pain with rapid appearance of swelling in the left forearm. Examination revealed swelling and marked tenderness in the left forearm just distal to the antecubital space—the area of the insertion of the biceps muscle at the tubercle of the radius and the deep fascia of the forearm. Diagnosis was made of sprain of the left biceps muscle at its radial insertion.

The only treatment suggested was daily application of a castor oil pack over the entire proximal half of the left forearm and the elbow to be left on all night long and worn as much during the day as possible. She was seen in three days and she stated that there had been a gradual disappearance of the swelling and pain. Examination showed all tenderness to be gone and all swelling subsided. She was discharged from care.

Response was rated excellent to single therapy.

CASTOR OIL PACK
INSTRUCTION SHEET

Instructions for use:

Prepare a flannel cloth which is two or three thicknesses when folded and which measures about eight inches in width and ten to twelve inches in length after it is folded. This is the size needed for abdominal application—other areas may need a different size pack, as seems applicable. Pour castor oil into a pan and soak the cloth in the oil. Wring out the cloth so that it is wet but not drippy with the castor oil (or simply pour castor oil onto the pack so it is soaked). Apply the cloth to the area which needs treatment. Most often, the pack should be placed so it covers the area of the liver.

Protection against soiling bed clothing can be made by putting a plastic sheet underneath the body. Then a plastic covering should be applied over the soaked flannel cloth. On top of the plastic place a heating pad and turn it up to "medium" to begin, then to "high" if the body tolerates it. It helps to wrap a large towel around the body to hold the pack snugly in place, using large safety pins on the towel. The pack should remain in place between an hour to an hour and a half.

The skin can be cleansed afterwards, if desired, by using water which is prepared as follows: to a quart of water, add two teaspoons baking soda. Use this to cleanse the abdomen. Keep the flannel pack wrapped in plastic for future use. It need not be discarded after one application, but can usually be used many times.

Footnotes

Chapter 1

1. Tierra, Michael, *The Way of Herbs*, Unity Press, Santa Cruz, Calif., 1980.

2. McGarey, William A., *Acupuncture and Body Energies*, Gabriel Press, Phoenix, Ariz., 1974, p. 8.

Chapter 3

3. Sugrue, Thomas, *There Is a River*, 3rd ed., Dell Publishing Co., Inc., New York, 1964.

4. Stearn, Jess, *Edgar Cayce — The Sleeping Prophet*, Doubleday and Co., Garden City, N.Y., 1967.

5. All extracts from the Edgar Cayce readings are identified by number (e.g., 1836-1, the first number representing the individual for whom the reading was given and the second number representing the number in the series given for that individual). The readings are available to the public in the A.R.E. Library in Virginia Beach, Virginia.

6. Millard, Joseph, *Edgar Cayce: Man of Miracles*, Neville

Spearman, London, 1961.

Chapter 5

7. Lee, Richard Y., *The Singular Sadness of Numerical Madness*, Continuing Education, Sept. 1983.

Chapter 6

8. McGarey, William A., *Edgar Cayce and the Palma Christi*, A.R.E. Press, Virginia Beach, Va., 1967.

9. McGarey, William A., *The Edgar Cayce Remedies*, Bantam Books, New York, N.Y., 1983.

10. *A Search for God*, Book I, A.R.E. Press, Virginia Beach, Va., 1942, 1970.

11. New English Bible, John 14:27.

12. Montgomery, D.W., "Castor Oil," *Journal of Cutaneous Disease*, 36:446, 1918.

Chapter 7

13. Grady, Harvey, "Castor Oil Packs: Scientific Tests Verify Therapeutic Value," *Venture Inward*, Virginia Beach, Va., July/Aug. 1988.

14. McGarey, *Edgar Cayce and the Palma Christi, op. cit.*

15. Gaddum, J.H., *Pharmacology*, 3rd ed., Oxford University Press, New York, 1949.

16. Montgomery, *op. cit.*

17. Cannon, W.B., *The Mechanical Factors of Digestion*, Longmans, Green & Co., New York, 1911, p. 51.

18. Goodman, L., and Gilman, A., *The Pharmacological Basis of Therapeutics*, The Macmillan Co., New York, 1941, pp. 801-829.

19. Starling, E.H., *Principles of Human Physiology*, 8th ed., C.L. Evans (ed.), Lea & Febiger, Philadelphia, 1941, pp. 224, 332-378, 675-676.

20. Schoch, A.G., "The Treatment of Dermatoses of Internal Origin with Castor Oil and Sodium Ricinoleate," *Southern Medical Journal*, 32: 326-328, 675-676.

21. Goodman, L., and Gilman, A., *op. cit.*, p. 801.

22. Ormsby, O.S., and Montgomery, H., *Diseases of the Skin*,

Lea & Febiger, Philadelphia, 1954, p. 129.

23. *Castor Oil and Chemical Derivatives*, Baker Castor Oil Co., Bayonne, New Jersey, 1962.

24. Novak, A.F.; Clark, G.C.; and Dupuy, H.P. "Antimicrobial Activity of Some Ricinoleic and Oleic Acid Derivatives," *J. Amer. Oil Chemists' Soc.*, 37:323-325, 1961.

25. Novak, A.F., et al., "Antimycotic Activity of Some Fatty Acid Derivatives," *J Amer. Oil Chemists' Soc.*, 39:503-505, 1961.

26. Schwartz, L., "Protective Ointments and Industrial Cleansers," *Med. Clinics of N. Amer.*, 26:1125-1210 (No. 4), 1942.

27. Srinivasan, T.M.; McGarey, William A.; Grady, H.T.; and Wisneski, L.A., *Immunomodulation Through Castor Oil Packs*, Fetzer Energy Medicine Institute (unpublished), A.R.E. Clinic, Phoenix, Arizona.

Chapter 8

28. Jarvis, D.C., *Folk Medicine*, Henry Holt & Co., New York, 1958, pp. 147-150.

Chapter 9

29. McDowall, R.S., *Handbook of Physiology*, 43rd ed., J.P. Lippincott Co., Philadelphia, 1964, p. 167.

30. West, E.S., et al., *Textbook of Biochemistry*, Macmillan & Co., New York, 1966, p. 1501.

31. Guyton, A.C., *Textbook of Medical Physiology*, 43rd ed., J. P. Lippincott Co., Philadelphia, 1964.

32. *Ibid.*, p. 45.

33. Wiggers, C.J., *Physiology in Health and Disease*, 2nd ed., Lea & Febiger, Philadelphia, 1937, pp. 263-275, 854.

34. Lewis, W.H., *Gray's Anatomy*, 23rd ed., Lea & Febiger, Philadelphia, 1936, p. 1164.

35. "Lymphatics' Role Stressed in Cardiovascular Disease," *Med. World News*, 7:100-101 (Jan. 21, 1966).

Chapter 10

36. *Blakiston's New Gould Medical Dictionary*, The Blakiston Co., Inc., New York, 1953, p. 243.

37. Starling, E.H., *Principles of Human Physiology*, 8th ed., C.L. Evans (ed.), Lea & Febiger, Philadelphia, 1941, pp. 224, 332-378, 675-676.

38. Netter, F.H., *Nervous System*, Ciba Pharmaceutical Co., Summit, New Jersey, 1962, pp. 80-100.

Chapter 11

39. Starling, E.H., *op. cit.*

Chapter 12

40. Starling, E.H., *op. cit.*

41. Strong, O.S., and Elwyn, A., *Human Neuroanatomy*, 5th ed. (Truex and Carpenter), Williams & Wilkins, Baltimore, 1964, pp. 131-145.

42. Chusid, J.G., and McDonald, J.J., *Corrrelative Neuroanatomy and Functional Neurology*, 8th ed., Lang Medical Publications, Los Altos, California, 1956, p. 154 .

43. Wiggers, *op. cit.*, p. 1164.

44. Starling, E.H., *op. cit.*, p. 224.

45. Reede, E.H., "Vegetative Nervous System," *J. Cut. Dis.* 36: 505-514, 1918.

46. Reede, E.H., *ibid.*, p. 506.

47. Starling, E.H., *op. cit.*, p. 368.

48. Goodman, L., and Gilman, A., *The Pharmacological Basis of Therapeutics*, 2nd ed., The Macmillan Co., New York, 1955, p. 1053.

49. Strong and Elwyn, *op. cit.*, p. 142.

50. Strong and Elwyn, *op. cit.*

51. McDowell, R.S., *op. cit.*, pp. 130-131.

52. Natter, F.H., *op. cit.*, p. 91.

53. Goodman and Gilman, *op. cit.*, p. 364.

54. Goodman and Gilman, *op. cit.*, p. 154.

Chapter 14

55. McGarey, William A., *The Edgar Cayce Remedies*, Bantam Books, New York, 1983.

56. See Part II, "Case Studies."

Index

A

incoordination and, 105-106
karma and, 99-100
lacteals and, 82, 87
on life purpose, 20-21
liver function and, 85
on love, 104-105
lymphitis and, 108
mental illness and, 151-153
on mystery, 29
nature of the body and, 101-103
on nausea, 106
nervous system and, 65, 75-76, 78-79
perception of body, 81
Peyer's patches and, 89-91
on physiology, 83-84
on pregnancy, 73
radiations and, 101-102
on snoring, 53
sympathetic nervous system and, 150-151
on vaginitis, 79
on vibrations, 32
view of illness, 56
Cayce, Hugh Lynn, 11
Cells
consciousness of, 158-160
drainage system of, 87
Central nervous system, 131, 132
Cerebral cortex, 131
Cerebral palsy, 58
Cerebrospinal nervous system, 133, 150
autonomic nervous system and, 109-114, 117, 127
conscious mind and, 164
sympathetic nervous system and, 91, 119, 123-125, 128, 151-156
Change, 23, 45
Chemical reactions, 63
Chest, packs over, 49
Chiropractic, 119
Cholecystalgia, 58
Cholecystitis, 58, 173, 182-184, 214
Cholinergic supply, 139
Christ Consciousness, 66
Chronic illness, 23-26, 64
Circulatory system, 110, 111, 200-201

Cleansing functions, 21, 184-185, 187
Coccyx, 94, 118-119, 152-153
Cocoa butter, 14, 78
Colds, 52
Colitis, 58, 207, 212-213
Colon, 57, 59-61, 83, 180-181, 190, 212
Colonics, 83
Communication, with body, 4-5
Conscious mind, 135, 154, 163, 164
Consciousness, 19-21, 131, 141
adventure in, 104
of cells, 111-112, 158-160
healing as an awakening in, 16-18
peace and, 168
purification in, 184-185
Constipation, 24, 58, 72-73, 159, 204
Contraceptive pills, 210-212
Coordination, 105-120, 145
Corns, 69
Courage, 161
Cranial nerves, 165
Creative activity, 45
Creative Forces, 3, 21, 23, 66, 102-103, 158, 201
Creative functions, 184
Cyst, 162, 209, 217
Cystitis, 206, 214

D

Dandelion, 2
Depression, 206-207
Dermatitis, 61-62
Detoxifier, 85
Diet, 95, 95, 107, 204. *See also* Food
Digestion, 82, 138
Dihydroxystearic acid, 62
Disease, 45
beginning stages of, 7
incoordination in, 105-114
Dizziness, 212
Doctors, *see* Physicians
Dorsal root, 118, 119
Dorsal spinal nerves, 124, 126-127
Dreaming, XVII-XVIII, 53, 95
communicating with body

through, 5
  Jesus in, 55
  physiological activity during,
    154
Duodenum, 58, 87
Dyslexia, 45

E

Ear problems, 49-52
Edema, 159, 172, 181, 212, 215
Edgar Cayce, *see* Cayce, Edgar
Edgar Cayce Remedies, The, 50
Efferent nerves, 132-133
Eicosanoic acid, 62
Electrical being, 102
Electrical vibration, 144-146
Electricity, 141
Electromagnetic radiation, 95, 102
Elimination
  autonomic nervous system
    and, 180
  castor oil and, 57, 189
  channels of, 39-40, 108
  emotions and, 200
  herb for, 2
  lymph and, 87, 93
Emollient properties, 63
Emotions, 53, 160-163, 200
  autonomic function and, 135
  disease and, 147
  disturbances of, 75-76
  effect on body, 7
  endocrine glands and, 137
  healing and, 96-120
  incoordination and, 114-120
Endocrine system, 85, 99, 127, 137,
    160-161
Endometritis, 215-216
Energy being, 102
Energy impulses, 130-131
Epigastric distress, 203
Epilepsy, 13-14, 58, 64, 90, 94
Esophageal spasm, 49
Exercises, 83
Eyes, irritation of, 68, 69

F

Faith, 17, 97, 142, 161

Fats
  lymph system and, 86
  in meals, 86
Fear, 161
Fecal impaction, 29-30, 80, 172, 180
Feet, 78
  aching, 44-45, 69
  stab wound, 217
  toenail fungus, 41
Fibrohematoma, 205-206
Fight/flight response, 137-138, 161
Fingernails, smashed, 39
Flannel cloth, 26, 219
Flatulence, 57
Folk medicine, castor oil in, 67-69
Food
  assimilation, 87, 88, 189
  emotions and, 200
  fats in, 86
  See also Diet
Foot, *see* Feet
Fracture, 217-218
Fungus, toenail, 41
Furuncle, 205

G

Gall bladder, 47-49, 57, 83, 98, 173,
    182-184, 204
Gallstones, 48-49, 57, 58
Ganglia, 133, 142-156
Gas, 24, 159, 180
Gastrointestinal complaints, 58, 72,
    213
Gastrointestinal tract, 73, 189
Genitourinary system, 73, 189
Gilman, A., 60, 62
Glands, 111, 160-163
Glycerol, 60
Glyco-Thymoline, 50
God, 201
  acceptance of, 6
  awareness of, 158
  Cayce on, 66, 100
  as Creative Force, 4, 18, 21
  faith in, 97
  manifestation of, 102-103
  material things and, 98
  meditative experience and, 65
  Temple Beautiful and, 95

Goodman, L., 60, 62
Guardian angels, 54
Gums, 167
Gynecological conditions, 185

H

Hair, 68, 210-211
Happiness, healing and, 8
Headaches, 77, 174, 186
Healing
    attitudes and emotions in, 96-120
    awakening of consciousness and, 16-18
    Cayce on, 22-23, 95-96
    change and, 23
    force, 19-34, 83
    happiness and, 8
    identifying, 165-168
    life force and, 158-160
    light, 50
    love and, 104-105
    massage and, 22
    parasympathetic nervous system, 179
    source of, 18
    touch, 67
    vibration, 55
Health
    incoordination in, 105-114
    Peyer's patches and, 89
Hearing loss, 51-52
Heart
    flow of blood in, 90
    lymph flow and, 92
Heart attacks, 154
Heat, 178
    contraindicated, 179-180
    relaxation and, 186
Heating pad, 26, 28, 84, 219
Hematoma, 39, 218
Hemoglobin count, 70-71
Hemoperitoneum, 209
Hepatitis, 47-48
Hernias, 21-22, 58
Hodgkin's disease, 58, 108, 117-119, 120
Hookworm, 58
Hormones, 99, 114, 160

Humor, sense of, 181-182
Hydroxyl groups, 62-63
Hyperactivity, 45-47, 65
Hypertension, 210-215. *See also* Blood pressure
Hysterectomy, 23-24, 159

I

Ileum, 87-88
Illness, 56
    understanding self and, 20
Imagination, 29, 128
Immune system/immunity, 64
    Cayce on, 74-75
    enhancement of, 27
    incoordination and, 108
    natural, 178
    Peyer's patches and, 88, 165
Immunizations, 81
Incarnation, moving through, 17
Incoordination, 105-120
Individual case, careful attention to, 19-20
Infection, after injury, 43-45
Inflammation, 57
    appendix, 178
    boil, 205
    dorsal area and, 127
    finger, 68, 173-174, 186-187
    vegetative nerve supply and, 126
Inhalations, 83
Injuries
    at birth, 39
    infections after, 43-45
Inquisitive spirit, 2
Intestines, 57, 85, 189
    obstruction of, 28, 29-30, 58, 172, 180-181
    See also Colon; Small intestine
Iron, 70
Irradiation, 60, 137
Itching, 61-62

J

Jarvis, D. C., 68
Jejunum, 87
Jesus, 4, 54, 55, 102, 171

Urinary wastes, 139
Uterus, 184
    fibroids in, 79
    hemorrhage of, 210

V

Vagina, 184
    discharge of, 215-216
Vaginitis, 79-80
Varicose veins, 36
Vegetative functions, 133
Verruca vulgaris, 209
Vertebrae, subluxation of, 119
Vibrations, 55
    castor oil creating, 30, 65, 167,
    179
    Cayce on, 32, 154
    changing, 23
    coordination of nervous sys-
    tems and, 154
    exercise on, 65
Violet ray, 74
Viscosity, 63
Visions, 154
Vitamins, 7-8
Vomiting, 97, 172-173, 213

W

Warts, 68, 209
Wisdom, 67
Wrist pain, 33

Y

Yeasts, 63